SHEILA LAMB & YEMI ADEGBILE

Infertility Doesn't Care About Ethnicity

Encouraging Tales About Conception Struggles

Dedicated to all Black, Asian, Indian and other ethnic woman around the world, who have, or are struggling to conceive. We see you. We hear you. You are not alone.

Contents

Acknowledgement

The idea for this book came during the Covid-19 pandemic, just after the Black Lives Matter protests. I, Sheila, have already published books that are collections of true-life stories about the emotional realities of the struggle to parenthood. However, I realised that although women and men from any culture experience similar emotions towards infertility and loss, those from certain ethnicities often also face judgement from their communities, and very often their own immediate families. This leaves them feeling more alone and isolated than their Caucasian counterparts, which takes a further toll on their mental health and well-being. This didn't sit comfortably with me, so I started researching, mainly on Instagram, to see if there were any Black, Asian, Indian and other ethnics women sharing their stories. There were. And they were very keen to share their experience in this book.

My thanks, firstly, go to Yemi, my co-author, who immediately came on board with this project as she works with ethnic women in the infertility field. Secondly, each contributor saw our vision for this book and kindly shared their experience to support you and raise awareness in cultures and communities where infertility and loss are taboo subjects. We appreciate each and every one of them, especially as we've never met but they now feel like family.

So, in alphabetical order: Abbe Meryl Feder @abbefeder, Aisha Balesaria @mindbodyrevival_coach, Anjulie @anjulies_mumoirs, Asia Cash @thefruitfulplace, Bimbola, Chi @makingbabyo_, Crystal-Gayle @4Damani, Gurinder Mann @adrugnamedhope, Kajal Pankhania @aurelias_wish, Karabo Zwane @hannah_youarenotalone, JO, Kezia Ashley Okafor @iamkeziaokafor, (Dr) Loree Johnson @drloreejohnson, Manjeet @fitspiration_fitter, Maria @mariainstaglam, Marise Angibeau-Gray @4memphys, Monique Farook @infertilityandmepodcast, @mysurrogatetwins, Nadine Gerin @nadinendoivf, Noni Martins @unfertility, Ola @thefertilityconversations and @fertilityconversations, Sally, Seetal Savla @savlafaire, Shannon Chapman @bellewithabump, Shayo O @naijafertilityhub, (Dr) Sierra Bizzell @ultimatefertilityconsultant, TJ Peyten @tjpeyten, Vaishali Bamania @jayas_star, Violet.

If you would like to connect with any of these lovely women, there's a 'Resources' section at the back of this book.

We've included some illustrations in the hope that they bring some comfort to you, and maybe give you a chuckle. Our illustrators are author, illustrator and IVF Mom Sheila Alexander (Instagram @sheilaalexanderart), and illustrator and author Phillip Reed, (Instagram @the_phillustrator, email philr@live.co.uk).

Cover illustrated by Best Page Forward.

Introduction

If you're reading this book because you're looking for support from other Black, Asian, Indian women, or women from other ethnicities, we're sure you'll find it within these pages – because dealing with infertility, fertility treatment, miscarriage, stillbirth, surrogacy or even finding yourself child-free after infertility, is anything but easy. All of these are taboo subjects around the world, even in the twenty-first century, which leaves women and men feeling very isolated and unsupported by their community.

Having been through infertility, IVF (In-Vitro Fertilization – where the egg and sperm are fertilized outside of the body), pregnancy loss and egg donation, I, Sheila, know how devastated I was when friends, family and colleagues were getting pregnant and having babies. It's so easy to let it take over your life; to forget who you are, to remember what you enjoy, to have fun, and still be the other half of a couple if you're in a relationship. Everything revolves around trying for a baby.

My wonderful co-author, Yemi, is a fertility nurse based in London, UK, and she says: "apart from working in a fertility clinic, I also support ethnic women and women of color who are living with infertility and going through fertility treatment."

Yemi and I both realized that it doesn't matter what a woman's skin color is or where she lives in the world, the emotions experienced in the struggle to conceive are the same. In addition to the anger, frustration, anxiety, depression and loneliness of infertility and loss, ethnic women also face long-held traditions regarding how families are raised, along with the importance of being a mother. This means that many women around the world, who don't know anyone else who's been through, or is going through, their situation, can feel isolated and so lonely. We don't believe it should be this way; no-one should feel alone when going through such a difficult time, and that's the reason why we're sharing the stories in this book.

We also realized that for women and men to receive better support from their immediate community, there must be an understanding of the emotional challenges of living with infertility and loss. In many cultures, the importance of women having children has been the norm since the beginning of time, so we know that changing deeply entrenched beliefs isn't going to happen overnight, but bringing about change has to start at some point – so why not now? We also mustn't forget that some women fortunately do receive loving support from their family and friends, despite the traditions of their culture.

For the stories to be authentic and unique, we approached women from different cultures and ethnic groups and told them about our vision for the book, and then asked if they wanted to be involved. Guess what? The answer was a unanimous, yes! Most of them aren't writers – their stories are in their own words with phrasing authentic to their culture, which will be recognizable if you're from that community. Situations they share haven't been embellished to shock you – their emotions are real, and their words come from the heart. Although all the stories are written by women, some do mention their husbands/partners as they, too, are affected by the struggle to become parents.

We're also grateful to the women who shared their feelings of bias because of their ethnicity, for example, when they weren't treated favorably in hospital having gone through miscarriage or premature labor. This is appalling, but sadly it's a known fact that not all healthcare professionals treat black women and women from ethnic minorities as considerately as they treat Caucasian women.

One of the passions behind writing this book was that studies show that, 'African American (AA) women are disproportionately affected by infertility in terms of prevalence, utilization of treatment, and access to care',(1) and that 'Even after adjusting for socioeconomic status, AA women aged 33–44 years were twice as likely to experience infertility in comparison to Caucasian American (CA) women'.(2) Even more concerning is that 'statistical trends have shown that infertility rates were increasing among AA women while simultaneously decreasing among CA women'.(3) And 'of the AA women who do seek infertility care, live birth rates after IVF are disproportionately lower than CA women'.(4) Shocking statistics.

The stories in this book are also from South Asian and Indian women who despite living in western society are still affected by their cultural traditions and face stigma and isolation. For Hindus, the religious need to have a son or a grandson stems from the tradition that the son performs the last rites during the father's death; an important symbol of rebirth. In conservative families, women aren't expected to work, but instead, remain at home to raise their family. Sperm and egg donation are frowned upon both culturally and religiously. If it is carried out, it's done so in secrecy, so that the child won't be told in case of repercussions for the entire family. In both the US and the UK, South Asian egg donors are in short supply.

In the greater Jewish community, laws need to be considered from the time of ovulation. For example, basal body temperature recording and ultrasound scans cannot be performed on the Shabbat (day of rest), and home ovulation test kits can be a challenge. During IVF, egg collection and transfer with regards to the mikveh (ritual cleansing) need to be considered. Often, a Rav (rabbi) will be involved in the IVF process. As with many cultures, there's often a stigma associated around infertility, with the couple often experiencing feelings of inadequacy which can lead to isolation and/or exclusion.

A lot of the women are not only sharing their stories in this book but have also decided to speak out and be seen because they know that there's nothing to be ashamed of. They have, or are still going through a life-changing event, and when this happens, many go on to find the strength and a desire to change their current situation. Often the husband is also supporting the 'trying to conceive' (TTC) community.

Some women have decided to remain anonymous. It doesn't

mean that they're ashamed or aren't as strong as the women openly sharing. Many Caucasian women also don't want to share their journey to motherhood. We're all different and that's okay.

It's also important to us that the stories cover the entire spectrum of trying to get pregnant and having a baby, so that people who haven't experienced a struggle know the realities. Their stories reveal:

- that IVF is not one-hundred per cent successful
- that after a woman has a miscarriage there are no guarantees that she'll get pregnant the next time and give birth to her baby
- that when her baby is stillborn, she won't ever 'get over it'
- that she is a mother regardless as to how her child was conceived, and
- that being child-free after infertility takes immense strength and courage.

As mentioned previously, although primarily we want the book to be a survival guide for women who are finding it a challenge to conceive, we also want it to be accessible to people who haven't experienced this struggle. One group is healthcare professionals: doctors, nurses, midwives, sonographers, embryologists, receptionists, as well as those practicing alternative therapies, counselors, and therapists, as well as religious and community leaders.

Every woman and man should be treated equally and respectfully. People need to stop pointing the finger of blame and instead ask how they can be supportive. Please feel free to connect with any of the women in this book; there is a 'Resources' section at the end with all their contact information. They'd love to hear from you and have the opportunity of supporting you.

Much love

Sheila & Yemi
   xx

References

1. Eichelberger KY, Doll K, Ekpo GE, Zerden ML. Black lives matter: claiming a space for evidence-based outrage in obstetrics and gynecology. Am J Public Health. 2016. https://doi.org/10.2105/AJPH.2016.303313; Seifer DB, et al. Trends of racial disparities in assisted reproductive technology outcomes in black women compared with white women: Society for Assisted Reproductive Technology 1999 and 2000 vs. 2004–2006. Fertil Steril. 2010. https://doi.org/10.1016/j.fertnstert.2009.02.084; Wellons MF, Lewis CE, Schwartz SM, et al. Racial differences in self-reported infertility and risk factors for infertility in a cohort of black and white women: the CARDIA Women's study. Fertil Steril; Shapiro AJ, Darmon SK, Barad DH, Albertini DF, Gleicher N, Kushnir VA. Effect of race and ethnicity on utilization and outcomes of assisted reproductive technology in the USA. Reprod Biol Endocrinol. 2017. https://doi.org/10.1186/s12958-

017-0262-5.

2. Eichelberger KY, Doll K, Ekpo GE, Zerden ML. Black Lives Matter: claiming a space for evidence-based outrage in obstetrics and gynecology. Am J Public Health. 2016. https://doi.org/10.2105/AJPH.2016.303313; Wellons MF, Lewis CE, Schwartz SM, et al. Racial differences in self-reported infertility and risk factors for infertility in a cohort of black and white women: the CARDIA Women's study. Fertil Steril. 2008. https://doi.org/10.1016/j.fertnstert.2007.09.056.

3. Seifer DB, et al. Trends of racial disparities in assisted reproductive technology outcomes in black women compared with white women: Society for Assisted Reproductive Technology 1999 and 2000 vs. 2004–2006. Fertil Steril. 2010. https://doi.org/10.1016/j.fertnstert.2009.02.084.

4. Eichelberger KY, Doll K, Ekpo GE, Zerden ML. Black lives matter: claiming a space for evidence-based outrage in obstetrics and gynecology. Am J Public Health. 2016. https://doi.org/10.2105/AJPH.2016.303313

Further Reflections

Learning about the infertility journeys of women in ethnic minority groups has been mixed with feelings of excitement and sadness. Sheila and I have collated all these experiences in the hope we can all learn about raising cultural awareness regarding these issues.

These narratives are the journeys, yearnings, heartaches, and joy of women and couples trying to conceive through In vitro fertilisation, known as IVF.

Not all of the tales have a happy ending; some are told from a point of resolution, either to move forward without a much-longed for baby or to pursue options such as adoption or fostering. But there's always something in every story for anyone who has either experienced infertility or knows someone who's currently going through it.

So why is infertility an issue in some cultures? Perhaps, because, there's still the stigma of women from the ethnic community bearing the brunt of judgement from close relatives and in-laws. The pressure to deliver children as soon as the marriage ceremony is over can often be overwhelming for a couple who may simply want to enjoy their new union without distractions; or they may wish to develop their careers first. Some cultures are still patriarchal in wanting a male heir to carry the legacy of the grandfather. This often happens when a family business has been handed down from generation to generation. Single women over forty who want a family fear being stigmatised because of the expectation to be traditional and have children with a man. The fear of the child being conceived by donated gametes (egg or sperm) is still a grey area that the ethnic community grapples with, therefore forcing those invested into secrecy.

Having looked after women and couples who are suffering from infertility, I've seen their anxiety while hearing their stories of silence, heated family discussions, unwanted involvement from in-laws, and feelings of isolation and shame.

The couples and single women who've eventually had a success-ful outcome after arduous rounds of fertility cycles are eternally grateful for their 'blessings', as they refer to them, and will forever cherish this experience. They are hopeful that their story will encourage others who are facing the same difficulties.

I hope their stories inspire you to never give up on your quest for a family in whatever form it takes. Culture is to be respected, yes, but there's also a need to understand that times have changed, and that time also embraces change.

Yemi Adegbile x

(In)Fertility Acronyms and Abbreviations

Before you start reading all the supportive stories, we thought it might be helpful to list the more common acronyms and abbreviations you'll come across - in this book, on social media, the internet, other books, blogs and articles - whilst on your journey to parenthood. It can be overwhelming at first and trying to work out what some of them stand for will have you scratching your head, but like all languages, it'll soon become familiar. If you want a full list of over 250, (yes, sorry, there are that many) acronyms/abbreviations, please feel free to download my free eBook here: https://www.mfsbooks.co .uk. And if you want in-depth, jargon-free explanations of medical and non-medical terms such as those listed below, Sheila's written *My Fertility Book: all the fertility and infertility explanations you will ever need, from A to Z*, which is available as an eBook and paperback from here: https://books2read.com/ u/mqoNd2

A

AF = Aunt Flo, After Flo, period, menstrual cycle

AFC = Antral Follicle Count

AMH = Anti-Mullerian Hormone

Angel baby = A baby lost during a pregnancy

B

BBT = Basal Body Temperature

Beta = hCG blood pregnancy test

BFN= Big Fat Negative pregnancy test

BFP = Big Fat Positive pregnancy test

C & D

CM = Cervical Mucus

DC = Donor Conception

D&C = Dilation & Curettage

DE = Donor Egg or Donor Embryo

DOR = Diminished Ovarian Reserve

E

EC = Egg Collection

ED = Egg Donor

Endo = Endometriosis

ER = Egg Retrieval

ET = Embryo Transfer

F

FET = Frozen Embryo Transfer

Frostie = Frozen embryo

FSH = Follicle Stimulating Hormone

Furbaby = pet cat/dog/other furry pet

H

hCG = Human Chorionic Gonadotrophin (pregnancy hormone)

HSG = Hysterosalpingogram

HyCoSY = Hystero-salpingo-Contrast-Sonography

I

ICSI = Intracytoplasmic Sperm Injection (a sperm is in injected into the egg to fertilise/fertilize it)

IUI = Intrauterine Insemination (sperm are placed in the womb to fertilise the egg)

IVF = In-Vitro Fertilisation/Fertilization (an egg and the sperm are placed in a petri-dish to fertilize)

L

LAP = Laparoscopy

LH = Luteinising/Luteinizing Hormone

LOR = Low Ovarian Reserve

M & O

MFI = Male Factor Infertility

OHSS = Ovarian Hyper-Stimulation Syndrome

OPT = Ovulation Predictor Test

OTD = Official Test Day - the day the clinic asks you to have a pregnancy test

P

PASP = Pregnant and staying pregnant

PCOS = Polycystic Ovarian Syndrome

PUPO = Pregnant until proven otherwise

R

Rainbow Baby = a baby born after a miscarriage, pregnancy loss of stillbirth

RPL = Recurrent Pregnancy Loss

S

Scanxiety = anxiety of ultrasound scans, especially after loss

SD = Sperm Donor

Stims = Refers to the medication to stimulate the ovaries to produce more eggs

T

TTC = Trying to Conceive

Transferversary = the anniversary day of your embryo/s transfer

Trigger shot = the injection that is done before egg collection/retrieval

TWW/2WW = Two-week wait until you do a pregnancy test

V & W

Vanishing Twin = the loss of one twin during a twin pregnancy

Wanda = the term used for an ultrasound scan

Letter to someone who's struggling to conceive

Dear lovely friend,

We want to give you a collective hug right now. You may not know anyone else who's struggled with infertility, miscarriage, stillbirth, or childlessness after infertility, but just because no-one has confided in you, you're definitely not alone.

Unfortunately, one in seven couples are infertile; this number could be much higher because many women don't seek help. Also, pregnancy loss is much more common than you probably think with one in four pregnancies ending in a miscarriage. Very few people expect their journey to parenthood to be long and difficult. So, when it doesn't happen easily for you, and you see friends fall pregnant seemingly quickly, it's understandable that you might feel frustrated, angry, sad, envious, stressed and anxious. These emotions are perfectly normal regardless of your age, religion or where you live in the world. You're fed up with waiting to become a mother and every baby announcement hurts more than the last.

It doesn't help when your friends and family start to lay on the pressure. Has anyone recently asked you, "When are you going to have children?" "You've been married for so long, what's the problem with you?" "You're thinking too much about it, just relax". You may just smile and murmur something unintelligible but respectful, when really you just want to run away before they see your tears. Everyone who's struggled to have a baby has been asked insensitive questions like these. And, it isn't fair or acceptable. If you're from a culture that has deep traditions around children and family, the constant reminders that you aren't yet a mother can leave you feeling ashamed and unworthy. But you have nothing to be ashamed of, and your life is as valuable as everyone else's.

If you spoke to every woman who wrote their experience in this book, that's exactly what they'd say to you, because they had these feelings too. They 'get it', but unfortunately your wider community doesn't. Not yet, anyway. You may have confided in a friend who you thought would be empathetic, only to be shocked that their words or actions were anything but. Understandably this may put you off speaking to anyone else, which leaves you feeling even lonelier.

But you don't have to manage all this on your own as there's fantastic support online which really does help – and you can dip in and out, as and when you feel the need. Women who are still struggling to create or add to their family are blogging, podcasting, doing webinars and Instagram/Facebook Lives, setting up Facebook groups and writing books about their experience. In the back of this book is a 'Resources' section, and most of the contributor's contact details are there if you want to connect. They would love to support you in any way they can ... and remember to tell them you read their story in this book.

If you've experienced a miscarriage, we are deeply sorry for your loss. Regardless of how many weeks pregnant you were, you already had hopes and dreams, and planned a future with your baby. Everyone's experience is unique, but from seeing those two pink lines or the words 'You're 2-4 weeks pregnant', you've already connected with your son or daughter. Maybe you only saw them as a tiny blip on the ultrasound scan or you were pregnant for many weeks, but now you've lost your long-awaited baby... we understand – it's impossible to prepare yourself for a loss like this.

How it happens is different for everyone, but how it feels emotionally is similar for many. The women in this book know what it's like to be excited about being pregnant, and then, moments later, to be told their baby has died. How do you deal with having your happiness snatched away so brutally? The first thing they'll tell you is that it isn't your fault. It wasn't because of something you did or didn't do. It wasn't because you ran for the bus or you had that extra cup of coffee. You couldn't have done anything to stop it from happening.

We're all different, of course, and some people will want to talk a lot about their experience, and others won't want to share. There's no right or wrong way; just do what feels right for you. If you've experienced an early miscarriage, people you confide in may struggle to understand why you're sad, and that's often because they've had no relationship with your baby. But, that cluster of cells was your dream, your future, and you

16

were already in love.

If your baby died later on in your pregnancy, people are usually more supportive, but often, due to feeling uncomfortable discussing miscarriage and the loss of a baby, they may not want to talk about your loss or your baby, and may even encourage you not to. We know you'll always want to talk about your baby, after all, you're their mother, so, why wouldn't you want to talk about your child?

Being child-free after infertility and loss is also a taboo subject in many societies, and even more so in ethnic communities because of the onus on having a family. Your own family may blame you for bringing shame on them if you don't have children. In truth, this is how a lot of women are living their lives. If this resonates with you, we recognize that your journey has been anything but easy and has likely affected your mental and physical health. We hope you don't feel shame because you absolutely shouldn't. Your life as a couple or as a single woman is as valuable as everyone else's. We know all women are not affected in the same way, i.e., facing stigma etc; many have a very supportive and open-minded family and in-laws which helps immensely.

By now, we hope that you can see that it isn't just you who's struggling on your path to parenthood. You're actually part of a club that no-one has asked to join, but when you're in it, you couldn't ask for more understanding, caring, and supportive members. After deciding to put this book together, we knew that when we approached women from various ethnic communities around the world and explained our vision, they would want to help their sisters. And they haven't disappointed, as they share, in their own words, how infertility, miscarriage, stillbirth, donor conception, surrogacy and being child-free after infertility, has encouraged them to be open about what they've dealt with. They are thinking of the future and how it will unfold for their own children or the children in their extended community. Please join us in applauding each and every one of them.

If you haven't told your family and friends about the challenges you're facing yet, because you don't know how to start the conversation, maybe it would help if you gave them a copy of this book and just tiptoed away, leaving them to read while you make a cup of tea or coffee. Or, if you've told family and friends, and they are consistently unsupportive, saying insensitive things, such as: 'just relax, it will happen', perhaps, give them a copy with some highlighted contributions that you think will help them be more empathetic.

We, and all the contributors, sincerely hope you find this book supportive. Many of the women said they found writing about their experience really helped them. Please, don't underestimate how infertility, having fertility treatment, and pregnancy loss affects your mental health. There's no shame in seeking professional support. What you're going through is incredibly hard, and it's now known that experiencing pregnancy loss can lead to post-traumatic stress disorder (PTSD). If your friend was dealing with PTSD, I'm sure you'd encourage them to seek support, so, it's perfectly okay for you to as well.

Lastly, if you know someone who needs to read other women's

stories on these topics, or who will better understand what it's like to struggle to have a family, please encourage them to read this book. You can also help others by leaving a rating or review on the online store you bought or downloaded this book from. Thank you.

Much love
Sheila & Yemi x

Letter to someone who hasn't struggled to become a parent

Dear friend,

Thank you so much for opening this book and taking the time to find out what it's really like for people in your culture and other cultures, who are struggling to start, or add, to their family.

Worldwide, one in seven couples are dealing with infertility, so it's extremely likely that a couple you know, and love, are going through this. The World Health Organisation (WHO) recognize infertility as a 'disease of the reproductive system', and as it takes a couple to make a baby, the cause can be a medical issue with either one or both. In fact, the latest statistics show that one-third of infertility cases are due to female medical problems, one third male medical problems, and in the other third, infertility is unexplained.

Two medical conditions that are common in African women are endometriosis and fibroids. Endometriosis is where tissue that is similar to the lining of the womb grows outside of the womb, such as the Fallopian tubes, the ovaries, and the bladder, causing pain that's often severe enough to affect the woman's lifestyle. Fibroids are benign tumours that grow in the wall of the womb and cause pain and often abnormal bleeding; they occur from the hormones estrogen and progesterone that women produce naturally. In South Asian/Indian women, there's a high incidence of polycystic ovary syndrome or PCOS. This is a condition where a woman's ovaries don't release an egg every month, which is thought to be caused by hormones.

Where men are concerned, the medical causes of infertility are abnormal sperm production, issues that may be due to undescended testicles, an unknown genetic defect, diabetes, mumps or enlarged veins in the testes. Also, sexually transmitted diseases (STIs), such as gonorrhea and chlamydia can, if untreated, cause genetic damage to the sperm. It's accepted in many cultures that the woman should be a virgin when she marries, although, this isn't the same for men.

So, it's clear that infertility is a medical condition rather than someone actively causing it. The stress of infertility has been compared in numerous articles to the stress of someone who has a cancer diagnosis, yet cancer patients aren't told that they're being punished for something they have or haven't done.

Some of what you read in the women's stories you may already be aware of because it's been this way for years in certain cultures. However, you probably won't appreciate how this struggle – infertility, fertility treatment, a different path to parenthood, miscarriage, stillbirth, and childlessness after infertility and loss affects your loved ones emotionally, every single waking moment. Honestly, it really is every minute of every day. Can you remember a time in your life when something really exciting was about to happen? Maybe you were going to university, you were getting married or were planning a fantastic holiday? Didn't you think about this 'thing' every minute? Did it take over your life? That's what it's like for someone who's struggling to have a baby or adding to their family. Only it's not exciting, but instead, anxiety making, stressful, frustrating, upsetting, depressing, and very lonely.

Let's consider the couple who are going through infertility and/or starting an IVF cycle, (In-Vitro Fertilization - where the sperm fertilizes the egg in a petri-dish in a laboratory). It's usually, though, not always, a busy woman who, as well as holding down a job, keeps a house running, looks after a young child and/or elderly relatives, and also has to squeeze in, often in secret from family and friends, the following:

- Hours and hours of medical research – trawling websites, reading books and articles, listening to podcasts, interacting on Facebook groups, and watching YouTube videos
- Researching the best nutritional supplements for herself and her partner
- Researching toxins in the house that could be affecting her/their fertility, then throwing it all away and replacing it with safe beauty/bathing/household products
- Navigating medical insurance forms if applicable
- Reading and replying to emails, taking and making phone calls with fertility clinic staff
- Diarizing appointments for investigations, scans, blood tests – for her and her partner
- Ordering medications and recording dosage along with the

exact times they're to be taken
- Giving herself the injections, or her partner/a friend may do this
- Dealing emotionally with family and friend's pregnancy announcements, gender reveals, baby showers and birth announcements
- Ensuring she's carrying out daily or at least regular, self-care for herself – journaling, meditation, exercise, mindfulness – to deal with the above
- Attending alternative therapy appointments such as acupuncture, reiki, reflexology, Emotional Freedom Technique (EFT), yoga
- Attending fertility counseling/coaching sessions
- Attending support groups
- If doing treatment overseas, researching flights, accommodation, and organizing currency.

Phew! And breathe! Quite a list on top of living a 'normal' life, isn't it? Oh, and she/they have likely tried superfoods, cut out things from their diet, drank disgusting concoctions, gone on holiday often, and got a furbaby (cat/dog/other furry animal). And she's put her legs in the air after sex, carried out numerous rituals, tried all the apps and prayed, a lot. She doesn't want to be told to 'just relax' or 'just adopt', and she definitely doesn't want to hear, 'it's meant to be'. Thank you.

The woman you know who's been married for a couple of years may not be doing IVF, but she may be mourning her babies that she lost early in her pregnancy. You may not be aware that she's been pregnant with her son or daughter; children that you would have met and loved. But for a reason that wasn't her fault, yes, not her or his fault, she miscarried their baby. Approximately, one in four pregnancies end in miscarriage. Shocking, isn't it? As soon as a couple see the word 'Pregnant' on a pregnancy test stick, they're planning their future life with this little being. At just four weeks pregnant, the baby's heart is already forming. At six weeks the heartbeat can be heard during an ultrasound scan – how amazing to hear a child's heartbeat when it's only the size of a grain of rice. At eight weeks the baby has arms and legs. Can you now see that a couple have lost their baby and why it's so devastating? Pregnancy loss before twelve weeks is very often a result of chromosome issues in the egg or the sperm – either too many or too few, or because either parent may have a genetic disorder. It's nobody's fault. Please remember that.

Pregnancy loss after twelve weeks, but before twenty-four weeks in some countries or twenty-eight in others, may be due to underlying health problems in the woman, such as diabetes, underactive or overactive thyroid gland, an immune issue that causes an increased risk of blood clots thus causing the placenta to fail, abnormalities with the womb or a weakened cervix. Or she could have caught an infection, had severe food poisoning, or be taking certain medicines for existing health conditions. But having an underlying medical condition doesn't mean she personally caused the loss of her baby. As you can imagine, she feels huge guilt and shame that it's her body that's broken, but there's no reason why she should feel or be made to feel this way. Other people who have medical conditions aren't made to feel guilty, and neither should she.

Miscarriage is NOT due to exercising too much, doing a job,

flying or eating spicy foods. Please read the above sentence twice.

The definition by the WHO of stillbirth is: 'a baby born with no sign of life at or after twenty-eight weeks of pregnancy.' In some countries, it's twenty-four weeks. The reason for the baby dying is often never known or it may be due to problems with the placenta or an infection. As you can imagine, the woman will blame herself. But she's definitely not to blame – but the 'what ifs?' and 'how did I not realize?' will always haunt her. You'll likely know that a couple in your family are expecting a baby and will, no doubt, be looking forward to meeting him or her. To hear that the baby has died is a shock – to you, to any siblings of the baby, and most importantly for the parents. You don't expect to lose a child yourself any more than the parents expected to lose their baby. They need your support, your love, understanding and most importantly, to acknowledge that their baby exists. They'd planned a future with this baby, had possibly started buying baby clothes and equipment and maybe, already decided on a name. The most caring thing you can do is call their baby by their name, let the parents talk about their baby whenever they want, and remember their baby in the future, just as you would a living child. They will be immensely grateful.

There are many different paths to parenthood that you may not be aware of. Parents can get pregnant with an egg from another woman, sperm from another man, an embryo made by another couple, or surrogacy; when another woman carries the baby (usually not from her egg), and gives birth. These different ways of becoming parents are down to the wonders of science

25

and are happening in countries around the world. Each miracle child is the same as every other child conceived without science – in fact, if you lined up ten children, you'd never be able to tell the IVF child or the child born via surrogacy from the naturally conceived child. And every child who's been conceived through science is loved by their parents.

Some couples go through infertility, multiple IVF cycles, recurring miscarriage, stillbirth, and unfortunately, never bring their baby home to show you. They remain child-free despite putting their heart and soul into trying to become parents. Please remember this when you're at a family gathering and you're about to ask a woman who doesn't have children, "When are you going to have children? You're not getting younger", or "Is there a problem why you don't have children yet?" What she'd prefer is to have caring comments, rather than intrusive questions or unhelpful advice. If you're not an extremely qualified fertility expert with loads of letters after your name, it's unlikely that you know more than she does. If she happens to mention something about why she doesn't have children, simply tell her you're there for her if she wants to talk or needs a hug. Treat her as you would like to be treated; if you wouldn't want to be bombarded with questions, don't do it to your daughter, daughter-in-law, sister, sister-in-law, cousin or best friend. And lastly, she and her partner aren't lucky that they don't have children because they can go on holiday whenever they want, have a tidy house, and can lie-in at the weekend. For a devastated potential parent, this isn't considered lucky.

As you read through these women's short stories, admire them for their honesty and for sharing their experience to help others know that they're not alone. Don't pity them or dismiss their emotions – they are grieving a life they thought they'd have. They would have loved to have made you a grandparent, an auntie or uncle, or given their child a sibling. They need your love and support, not for you to be embarrassed because of what others will think.

If you know someone who'd find support from the shared stories or who will better understand what it's like to struggle to have a family, please encourage them to read this book. And help others by leaving a rating or review on the online store you bought or downloaded the book from. Thank you.

Much love
  Sheila & Yemi x

Tackling cultural taboos in infertility

My fertility journey started almost eleven years ago, long before the creation of Instagram or Facebook fertility accounts that can now be used as a source of information, support and community. It was a very lonely time.

After I got married, I felt increasing pressure to have a child when the same question would constantly arise at community gatherings: "so, when are you having a baby"? Although these questions were painful, I was mindful that I had to reply with respect to the elders from my community, no matter how inappropriate the interrogation. A scenario, I'm sure, a lot of people reading this can relate to.

We 'tried' for two years with no success. Eventually, a thorough laparoscopic investigation revealed that I had stage 4 endometriosis; this culprit was the primary cause of my infertility. My diagnosis came as no surprise – for years, doctors had dismissed the pain, fatigue and bleeding as 'bad periods', but I always knew it was much more than that. The next decade was dominated by fertility treatment: over eleven unsuccessful IVF attempts, one failed IUI (intra-uterine insemination), and four miscarriages. Trying to conceive completely ruled my life for a very long time. It was a difficult journey that affected my relationships as well as my mental and physical health. It left me heartbroken. However, with real courage and determination, I eventually got to a place of healing and acceptance of my current, childfree-after-infertility life.

Regardless of race or community, we are all casualties of infertility and the stigma and shame that can be associated with it; however, the shame and stigma are even more prominent within South Asian and Middle Eastern communities because of tradition and culture.

Contrary to popular belief, there's no one-size fits all when it comes to how a person chooses to embrace their culture. Each country has its own unique heritage which can include different languages, religions, customs and societal norms. Because of this, each person's infertility experience will vary. While I've met both South Asian and Middle Eastern women who've felt no stigma at all regarding their fertility issues, I've also met many who've faced huge challenges. As a person who's half South Asian, I was incredibly fortunate to have a supportive network of family and friends. Even so, there were many times when I felt under pressure from the wider South Asian community.

Why is there so much stigma in our communities regarding infertility?

Stigma exists because of the deep-rooted cultural narrative – family is the 'centre' of everything. In many communities, having children is the default once married, and a pregnancy is expected to be announced immediately. There can also be added pressure on individuals from larger families to follow in the footsteps of their parents or grandparents.

Misinterpreted religious beliefs also play their part, with some perceiving infertility as a spiritual trial and part of God's will, rather than a medical condition. Couples are usually encouraged to pray harder, instead of seeking medical treatment.

The pressures associated with infertility can also be disproportionately placed at the feet of women. A woman is seen as the child-bearer in South Asian and Middle Eastern culture, and when pregnancy doesn't happen, the assumption is usually that she is at 'fault', causing deep shame, embarrassment and misplaced guilt. Fertility is a huge responsibility and burden placed on us as women; this is despite research that male factor infertility represents forty to fifty per cent of all infertility cases.

Infertility is just one taboo – baby loss, chronic illness and divorce still remain highly stigmatised, even in the 21st century.

The good news is that more and more South Asian and Middle Eastern women are sharing their journeys on social media, helping them to feel less alone. However, Muslim women are often unwilling to show their faces, and many still choose to remain anonymous – probably for fear of others finding out.

The deep issues concerning attitudes around infertility and its causes, and the stigma associated with it, are generally misunderstood, even in wider society. Therefore, tackling the taboo of infertility is much harder to combat within South Asian and Middle Eastern communities because of the added layers of tradition and culture.

How can we change the stigma surrounding infertility in our communities?

We need to work together to help shift the cultural mentality surrounding fertility. Infertility must be recognised as a medical condition, just like any other. We need community and religious leaders to speak openly about the modern-day challenges that couples face, including being unable to conceive. The focus must be on supporting couples/individuals by showing empathy for the difficulties they face, whilst encouraging families not to pinpoint blame as this only leads to more pressure. Couples/individuals need to be encouraged and supported by their families to seek medical help if they wish, and to attend support groups or therapy if needed. We need to change the narrative that infertility isn't caused by something someone did or didn't do, including, 'not praying hard enough'. We need to stress that not being able to conceive is nothing to be ashamed of and having a life without children can be equally fulfilling and of equal value. I am living proof that a childfree life can be an amazing one. We also need to be mindful that the modern-day South Asian person, for example, will have very different views from their grandparents, therefore, how they choose to live their lives in current times should be respected.

What can we all do?

· Work with us: we need bloggers with a larger following to amplify our voices so that we can widen the debate and get our stories heard.

- Representation matters: we need fertility clinics to have better representation in images and stories because they're still very focused on the typical Caucasian family. This makes people reluctant to seek help when they don't feel as though the narrative includes them.
- Build trust in healthcare: there's huge mistrust that needs turning around. People facing infertility are more likely to seek help if they feel as though they're not being dismissed or judged because of their cultural beliefs.
- Lastly, it really is all about inclusion: include us, it's so important. All our stories matter and for those suffering from shame, embarrassment and isolation, an image or story that reflects our lived experiences can make all the difference.

Aisha Balesaria @mindbodyrevival_coach

I'm sorry, there's no heartbeat

"I'm so sorry, there's no heartbeat..." Six words that changed my life forever.

At twenty-three plus three weeks pregnant on Monday 27th May 2019, I woke up as usual at around 6.30 a.m., but there was something unusual about this particular morning ... I couldn't feel my baby moving. At first, I didn't worry too much, innocently assuming that after a hot cup of tea and some breakfast, I'd soon feel the familiar kicks, but as my day unfolded, this didn't happen.

It was a gloriously sunny day on this perfect May bank holiday; I had my hair half up in a clip, wearing a khaki green jumpsuit that proudly displayed my growing bump. We had a lovely day planned, meeting family for brunch in the gardens of a beautiful pub, and I was so looking forward to catching up with them and making the most of the extended weekend. When we arrived, there was a band playing along with face painting for the children; I became lost in the happiness of my day. We ate, we drank, and we laughed until our bellies hurt. My eldest son, Virráe, ran around, doted on by everyone, and as I glanced at my watch, thinking it must only be about midday, I was shocked to see that it was already 3.00 p.m. My heart sank when I realised that I'd still not felt any movement. I remember feeling scared. I could feel my heart racing and my skin getting hot – that sick panic-stricken feeling that you only get when something is completely out of your control – what was so wrong that my baby hadn't moved?

I discreetly managed to let my husband Nik know something wasn't right, and I recall him saying "why didn't you tell me sooner?" I couldn't answer him; I couldn't even think; the only thing I could feel was fear.

Our family lovingly pleaded with us to stay longer, completely unaware of what was really going on, but somehow, we managed to paint a smile on our faces, make our excuses and leave. The journey to the hospital was silent and still, I couldn't hear a sound. It seemed even the birds had stopped tweeting; perhaps, they knew, too. I stared out the window clutching my stomach. I knew in my heart that something was very wrong with our baby, and I suspect Nik did as well.

I spent what felt like hours pacing the hospital waiting room; it was as though the clock just wasn't moving. My name was finally called, and we were ushered into a room. The midwives chattered away, telling me that my baby was just causing mischief. I couldn't even utter a word in response, I just let my head fall back as I shut my eyes and prayed. After multiple nurses failed to find my babies heartbeat, I was struggling to control my emotions, but with Virráe in the room, I had no choice but to remain calm. I paced up and down, clenching my fists as the hot tears raced down my cheeks. The voice inside my head was screaming that my baby had died, and I wanted to scream back and make this whole nightmare go away. After an agonising wait, the on-duty consultant came in and confirmed the devastating reality that was to change our family forever – the voice inside my head was right ... my baby had died!

My body gave way and I fell to the floor. Two midwives caught me, and as they did, an unrecognisable scream left my mouth. Tears poured from my eyes, and as I looked at them, my face pleaded with them to fix this. They, in turn, looked back, tears streaming down their cheeks, and I knew then, as we spoke with our eyes, that this could never be fixed, and nor could I. Unable to walk, I was wheeled into another room for one final scan. I recall the midwives telling me not to worry about Virráe, and asking whether or not he was allowed biscuits. Whilst so much of what happened is a haze, my brain has the most insignificant moments of that day etched in precise detail. Little did I realise at the time, but the trauma was already leaving a trail of destruction in its wake. I was unsure of how to process the mass of information that I'd nodded my way through with the senior midwife. There wasn't one word that I remembered she said, only that was she was kind, and when I was with her, I felt safe.

As we left the hospital, once again in silence, everything felt like an out of body experience. Was this really happening to me, or was I about to wake up from a nightmare? I watched my son run ahead of us in the empty car park with face paint smeared down his cheeks. When the midwives had kindly taken care of him, they gave him some gloves and a plastic apron to take home and he still had these on. He looked ridiculous, but I remember thinking if anyone could see us now, they'd never know the reality of just how dark our world had become. I remember saying that I needed to call my mum, and Nik telling me he would take Virráe to pay for the ticket to give me some privacy. This was quite possibly the hardest phone call I've ever made in my life – how do you explain that your baby has died, but that you're still carrying them in your womb, and that you still have to give birth, that you have to plan a funeral? How do you explain something that simply doesn't happen to you? Somehow, I did, and so my devastating journey of loss and life afterwards began.

Three days after learning my baby had died, I gave birth to a perfect little girl. The labour was painful and intense, but it was beautiful. Our daughter silently entered this world, and when she was placed in my arms, her beauty took my breath away. How could a child so utterly perfect be lifeless? Her face was heart-shaped like mine, and I traced her soft skin with the tips of my fingers; if I close my eyes, I can still feel her now. She had lips that were as red as a rosebud, a perfectly shaped nose, and eyes big enough to get lost in. We named her Aurelia, meaning 'The Golden One'. I looked at her, and then I looked to the sky, and I willed us to defy science; I willed her chest to start moving, and I willed for life and not death, but sadly my prayers weren't answered.

We spent the next few hours with her; I dressed her, held her and kissed her. I read her a bedtime story and just lay watching her and taking lots of photos that I will cherish forever. She somehow gave me the strength to enjoy this time. I felt so proud like any new mum, and it felt lovely to potter about our hospital bedroom just knowing she was there. We invited the grandparents to come and meet her, and their eyes were brimming with pain, but also with pride. I think they drew strength from seeing Nik and I so united, and of course, seeing their beautiful granddaughter. We decided that we wanted to let her go before the day was over. I somehow didn't feel able to go through the night with her; I didn't want to give myself false hope that she would, by some miracle, wake up and that I'd be able to take her home. Just before midnight, I read Aurelia a book called: *Guess How Much I Love You* ... to the moon and back of course, and I kissed her goodnight for the first and last time, and then she was gone. Nik and I climbed into bed in the bereavement suite, and for a while, we just held one another in complete silence, but eventually, we turned away from each other to be alone, and for the first time in days, we slept.

The grief was overwhelming, and it took over every part of my mind, body and soul. It was there, around every corner and behind every door, I couldn't escape it. It felt like a tennis ball in a jam-jar, all-consuming with no space for anything else to move around. I couldn't make sense of life; I only knew that the old me had died with my daughter and that I had no idea who the new me was. The only thing that kept me going was planning Aurelia's funeral; it kept my mind busy, so busy that I worried about what I'd do with myself afterwards. It was the last thing I'd ever be able to do for our daughter, so I had to put my body, mind, and soul into it.

I worried that there would be pressure from family to do things a certain way or invite certain people, and in my mind, I'd already become defensive about this. Whilst I was raised within a South Asian family, and also lived with my grandparents, my parents had always been extremely liberal. They taught me to be respectful yet encouraged me to challenge them when I thought differently, to ask why, and to be independent. All the girls that married into our family were treated like daughters and accepted for being them, and so I grew up thinking that this was what married life was like. When I happened to fall in love with an Indian boy, also from a South Asian family, I naively thought nothing much would change, and I would simply slot in, but in reality, life became very different. I faced some particularly challenging situations in the earlier years of my marriage; my confidence was slowly and painfully torn apart until it had completely diminished. Far from being accepted, I was instead, expected to understand my place in the family, and as a married woman, there was a very clear sense of control over what I should and shouldn't do. Decisions were made based on what others would think, or what would make the family 'look good' with little regard for wellbeing or happiness. The line between respect and control were so blurred, it was almost impossible to tell the difference. In the end, I had a nervous breakdown, but after seeking help, I regained my strength and began to stand up to the control, to call it out, and to do what felt right for me again. Perhaps this journey of self-discovery was needed so that I would have the strength to face other battles that life had waiting for me.

Within the Hindu culture, it is said that if a child passes before the age of five, then their bodies should be buried and not cremated, but I simply couldn't bear the thought of Aurelia's little body lying underground. Nik felt the same, and we instinctively knew that we wanted to have her cremated. We had full support from everyone on both sides of the family and were encouraged to do what felt right for us. This was so refreshing, and almost a shock to the system, as it was the first time we were being treated like adults with our decisions respected without interference.

After worrying about who to invite to the funeral, we decided that we only wanted a handful of our closest friends and family there ... that absolutely no one on the guest list should be there because of their status; it had to be because of a personal relationship with us. With this in mind, there were individuals who we consciously chose not to invite because of the way they'd treated me in the past, and I was shocked that this decision wasn't challenged. For once, the focus was truly about supporting us, and not what others would think of our choices. It seemed that there was no longer an expectation for us to make decisions based on what 'looked good', or what would please our elders, in fact, I'd go as far as saying that there was no expectation at all.

On the day, I woke up with my stomach in knots, and my eyes heavy from days of crying. I was starting to feel defeated, or perhaps, I was already defeated ... I didn't know. I didn't know anything anymore. I tried to put on some makeup, but nothing could mask the grief, and so I wiped it all off again. One less thing to worry about, I thought. Time seemed to have stood still as the rain poured from the sky as if even nature was mourning my little girl.

The funeral car arrived, and there inside was the tiny little coffin that held my baby. I closed my eyes and pictured Aurelia just as

39

I'd dressed her the day before, adorned in pink and tucked up tight with a few special things next to her. Nik and I sat either side of her, and I couldn't help but think that this wasn't how the first car journey with our daughter was meant to be. We both placed our hands on top of her coffin, and I think in a way, we just wanted to make the most of having her near us.

We arrived at the crematorium, and I could see the last of our family and friends making their way in … it all suddenly felt so real, too real. I got out of the car and as I composed myself, Nik wrapped his arm around my waist, and when I looked up, the funeral director was holding my daughter in her arms. Tears once again filled my eyes and as she placed her coffin in my arms, with Nik beside me, I carried her for the very last time.

The weeks that followed Aurelia's funeral were a bit of a blur; they came and they went. I went back to work and suddenly it was the end of the year. How had I survived seven months after her death? 2019 was the year that I came to know the type of love I'd only ever dreamt of, for it was meant to be the year that I'd completed my family. When Mother Nature put me on a different path, I came instead to know a harrowing pain that I didn't know could co-exist so beautifully with such profound love.

I lost my faith in life and its plans for me, and I learnt firsthand just how ignorant the human race could be. And when I was forced to look a little closer to home, I was saddened to experience how deep-rooted the stigma of stillbirth and baby loss remains in the South Asian community. It's the reason why so many feel the need to keep quiet, to grieve alone, and to suffer in silence. People are made to feel this way because others find it uncomfortable. That's exactly why I will keep talking. And I will shout as loud as my voice will carry, for me, for Aurelia and for every single person that feels they can't. Although she took not one breath, Aurelia opened up the eyes of those around us, specifically some of our elder family members. She made them see that the opinions of others do not matter, but that the well-being of loved ones does. She helped them realise the need to recognise and validate feelings and emotions, of talking and being open, but of also showing emotion themselves. She broke down the walls and brought us all closer together. She helped me to become accepted and to be confidently and unapologetically me. If losing Aurelia has taught me anything, it's that love, kindness and honesty can change the world. Her short but powerful life has reminded me that there is beauty in everything, and always something to be grateful for.

Kajal Pankhania @aurelias_wish

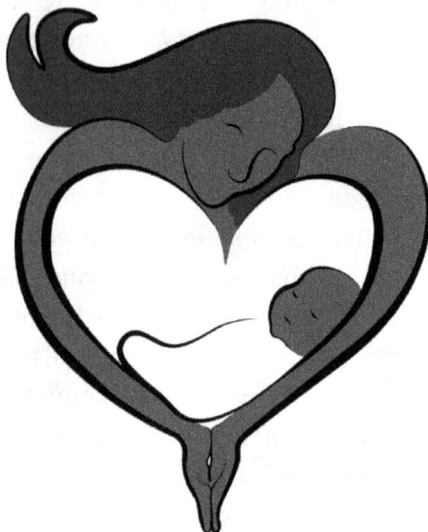

You carry your baby in your heart

The sole purpose of a woman is not motherhood, nor a man, fatherhood

Each person's experience is different within every culture. The information highlighted here is based on my own circumstances and that of others I've been in contact with. For some, their experience might be more successful in terms of outcome than those mentioned, and for others, it could be far worse. For a country with over two hundred million people, there's a lot of diversity, and everyone's story is unique.

In general, society expects that everyone will aspire to become a Mum. There is no question about whether you would like to have kids or not; it's assumed. There are expected stages throughout our lives – go to high school, go to university, get a job, get married and have children, raise your children and so on. As the different milestones are what are often promoted and spoken about, people experiencing difficulty in attaining them can often feel some form of shame/stigma and pressure to work harder.

If you do get married, you will often hear friends and family comment about their plan to return to your home in nine months to celebrate the birth of your child or children. This naturally can create a level of pressure on the couple.

If the couple doesn't have a child within one to two years, it's not uncommon for people to make comments such as: "What's taking so long?" "What are you waiting for?" "You aren't getting any younger." On the extreme end, some might tell the woman of the need to hurry and have a baby to prevent the husband from having one outside the marriage. Again, the assumption is that women are the ones that have the problem if a child isn't forthcoming.

There still needs to be awareness about male factor infertility, awareness about infertility and the impact it can have on the individuals and their wellbeing. Some comments from family and friends – though often well-intended – can add to the already stressful situation, so, there's a need for awareness on how to support people with infertility in terms of what and what not to say.

In addition, some people in your community might also question if you're actually serious about achieving the goal of having a baby, especially if it appears, you're unbothered about the delay in conceiving. If you're living your best life and having a great time, often attending parties and events, it's not uncommon for people to wonder out loud why you're still socialising instead of focusing your energy on achieving the goal of having children.

There needs to be more awareness about the fact that the sole purpose of a man and a woman isn't motherhood or fatherhood. Yes, many of us aspire to become mums, but some women

THE SOLE PURPOSE OF A WOMAN IS NOT MOTHERHOOD, NOR A MAN,...

might not want children and that should be okay. And those that aspire to become mums might not be able to achieve that goal. Regardless of one's parental status, everyone's life is worth celebrating and everyone should be made to feel like they matter and are worthy of a beautiful life.

Ola @thefertilityconversations and @fertilityconversations

What not to say (pregnancy loss)

This excerpt is based on two blogs called: 'What Not to Say' and 'Helpless'.

If you know someone who is grieving, and you think "I don't know what to say" – just **try**. Because just imagine if everyone took your approach. Where would your grieving friend be?

Alone ...

One of the things that has hurt me the most in this entire journey is the people who've said nothing. The friends and family and colleagues who ignored my pain, who ignored my children. I have lost three babies. I am grieving. If grief is uncomfortable for you, imagine what it's like for the person going through it: if something is hard to do, perhaps it's all the more worthwhile.

So, what's the one thing you shouldn't say to someone who's grieving? Nothing. I understand that it's impossible to find the perfect words, but we can try to educate ourselves in order to avoid the offensive ones. What starts with sympathy could easily end in empathy.

It's important for me to note that causing inadvertent offence transcends race, religion, culture – no one section of society has the monopoly on this – there's no pattern to the people who've managed to upset grieving parents in the baby loss community.

I am a British Indian, married to a white Christian. We straddle two cultures and both families have managed to upset us. On my husband's side, it's his family's silence that I will never forget – the many things left unsaid. On my side, it's the (sometimes advertent) offence caused by the unhelpful comments.

I know that it's difficult knowing what to say – it's now seven months since our daughter Summer passed away, and I too, have to pause, and really think before speaking to someone who's living through baby loss. It still doesn't come naturally to me either – but I just want you to understand how some platitudes sound when you're on the receiving end of them. So, please, despite the tone, don't take this as an attack, rather an insight into how we can help each other and what might work better going forwards.

The Definite Statements
"It will happen for you"
"It just takes time"
"You will have a baby one day"

I understand that it's well-meaning, but you don't know this for certain. There are no guarantees in life; sometimes it doesn't work out. Does your certainty bring you comfort? Because I'm sorry, try as I might, it doesn't bring me any. None. Often it just adds an additional layer of either anger or pressure, and definitely, sadness.

My entire experience of pregnancy is about loss. Has that sunk in? Do you understand how it's all ruined now? I was confident it would work out the first time. I'm never going to be moving forwards. There's no certainty here, not for me.

I know that what's being said all comes from a position of hope, so, please, just say that. Say "I believe it will happen for you" or "I hope you'll be able to bring a baby home one day", because the only thing that any of us can offer, is hope. Diminished as mine is.

The Success Stories

"My friend/sister/aunt had five miscarriages and now she has two children!"

"I know someone who went through IVF and then she had a child naturally afterwards!"

I've lost count of the 'success stories' I've heard since I miscarried. Granted, this isn't the same for everyone, but I want to playback what I hear when the above is said. Firstly, I hear FIVE miscarriages. I don't hear the happy ending ... I hear FIVE. I think: *I've had three miscarriages; I can't have two more! I can't keep doing this. It's cruel: to me, to the babies. Five!*

Secondly, illogical as it may sound, when I hear a success story, I just think it depletes the odds for me. I think: *good for them, but some people never have children, so if they've been successful, that means my chances of having one just fell.*

When you're stuck in your personal nightmare, other people's happy endings don't help much. Instead, I suggest just listening. Listen to their memories of their babies and their experience, without trying to offer silver linings or solutions.

The Cultural Curiosities

"Everything happens for a reason"
"Your baby was too pure for this world"
"Do you think you exercised too much?"

In my husband's family they focus on silence and 'less is more', but I sometimes feel that my family think they have a license to say whatever they like. It's part of the Indian culture – for the elders to be given free rein, regardless of the feelings of others. I'm not sure which is worse: the silence or the verbal diarrhoea?

I'm lucky that my Indian family is not particularly 'traditional' or as stereotypically overbearing as one might think, but there are notable differences from my white-British in-laws. For example, none of my in-laws would dream of suggesting that I was exercising too much, let alone actively put that question to me, as my own family did. Thanks, guys, that's really helpful, suggesting that I was the cause of my baby's death! I exercise regularly, I eat well, I have a perfect BMI; because of this, I have time and again been labelled a low-risk pregnancy by my medical team. In the Indian culture, however, exercising when pregnant is taboo, and instead, over-eating is actively encouraged – which is laughable really, because then when you later struggle to lose the baby weight, they'll be sure to comment on that too.

49

One other thing that people in my culture have been inclined to do, is to link my baby's death to some higher purpose, suggesting that they were somehow chosen for this. Although this may have brought comfort to the older generation, I've found that it resonates much less with the younger, less religious cohort. Do you realise that you're implying that my babies are better off somewhere else, other than with me? That somehow you deserved your children, but that I did not? No, not everything happens for a reason. Sometimes the proverbial just hits the fan, no reason required.

One bereaved parent, who's a Muslim, told me that in her faith, they believe that time behaves differently in the afterlife and that one thousand years on earth is the equivalent to one day in heaven. That means that our babies will see us again before they even know it – that's the type of religious statement that may bring comfort to the bereaved. Note the subtle difference: one excuses the loss, the other kindly acknowledges it.

The Glancing Forwards
"At least you can conceive"
The funeral will bring closure"
"You can move forwards now"

Funerals do not bring closure; I'm starting to wonder if anything will. I don't think so. When something dies – a person, a friendship, a relationship – it's never placed in a box, tied up with ribbon and put away neatly. In fact, it's more like *well, that was unexpectedly sh*t. I now have this huge hole in my life. No reason for it that I can fathom, but there it is.* There's no way or plan to get around it, it just is. And I guess you just have to learn to live with it. That's not gaining closure, or moving forwards, it's just waking up every day in a world which looks and feels quite different all of a sudden.

So, please, be careful about being dismissive of the babies who've passed. Getting pregnant again doesn't compensate for the past loss or make any of it okay. It's not about getting a replacement baby; it's about wanting the ones we've lost.

Having read this back, the above may all seem obvious, but you'd be surprised at how commonly these statements are made. Sometimes the comments land better than at other times, for example, when a doctor says, "this will happen for you, I've seen it happen" – that may give comfort.

Still, at least you now have a glimpse of how sometimes the best-intended remarks can unintentionally fall short of their goal.

Anjulie @anjulies_mumoirs
  Link to blogs www.Mumoirs.co.uk

Infertility trauma is racial trauma

Based on the blog: Infertility Trauma is Racial Trauma

I write this blog as a Black woman, a Black therapist, and a Black female who's a member of 'The Infertility and Grief Communities.' Being part of these different communities has often left me feeling disjointed. I can speak about my experiences of racism with my black community, and I can talk about my pregnancy losses with my infertility community – but I struggle to find ways to marry the two worlds. Years ago, in a conversation I had with a friend who was also a professor of social justice issues, I shared how my experience of racism impacted my fertility. But without sound scientific evidence, the discussion ended there. I could never fully process this with the members of my infertility community. The overwhelming majority of professionals, therapists, and coaches couldn't comprehend the depths of my racial experience which created another barrier.

The Intersection where infertility trauma and racial trauma meet

Being a part of the infertility community can bring about feelings of isolation in its own way, much like my experience within the racial community. However, I never fully conceptualized or owned the impact that racism and racial injustices have had on my reproductive health until recently.

I know the trauma of infertility. I've suffered four pregnancy losses, and I endured five mini-IVF (in-vitro fertilization), rounds with only a chemical pregnancy to show for it. The hormones and repeated losses threw me into a world of grief and isolation. When I began seeing social media posts about infertility trauma without any reference to what was happening within the Black community, I became even more triggered.

Infertility and other fertility issues have long been considered something that only impacted white people. Stereotypes around Black female fertility portray us as hyper-fertile, thus having no problem procreating. It's one of the reasons that discussing fertility issues is so challenging within the Black community. Assuming the validity of these stereotypes' delays many within our community from seeking help, while some choose not to access services at all. If you're working with people of color, particularly Black women and men, you need to understand the intersection between racial trauma and fertility trauma.

Discussing issues of race is already a challenge. But discussing intersectionality is even harder. Understanding the connections between racial trauma and fertility trauma is essential to understanding the USA's history with slavery and discrimination.

Infertility and racism: a complicated history
Born in 1813 in Lancaster County, South Carolina, Dr. James

Marion Sims was considered a pioneer in women's reproductive health, having developed tools and surgical techniques used today. He is regarded as the "father of modern gynecology." Dr. Sims was also a slaveholder, and he conducted research and experimental procedures on enslaved women, without anaesthesia. Since they were viewed as property and devoid of human rights, these women couldn't give consent or take ownership of their bodies. His decision to operate on enslaved women was informed by his assumption that they didn't feel pain. This concept still exists in the medical community as confirmed in a 2016 study conducted at the University of Virginia. His work is part of a long history of medical apartheid, which includes the Tuskegee syphilis experiment and the stolen cells of Henrietta Lacks, that have generated millions of dollars for the medical community without any compensation to her or her family.

Racism in the research

In 2019, the American Society for Reproductive Medicine (ASRM), noted that racial disparities in fertility care continue to exist. Their findings are compelling and validating:

"The success rate, measured as the ratio of live births per ART (Assisted Reproductive Technology) cycle, was lower for Black women, and the miscarriage rate was higher. Using statistical methods, the researchers found that race was an independent factor related to a live birth, even when controlling for age, BMI (Body Mass Index), previous pregnancy, and etiology of the infertility."

Subtleties around race and white privilege extend into how a diagnosis is made. The difference in the rates at which African-

American women were misdiagnosed with pelvic inflammatory disease (PID – an infection that develops in the female reproductive organs), and sexually transmitted infections (instead of fibroids – non-cancerous growths that develop in or around the womb, or endometriosis – tissue similar to the lining of the womb which attaches to other areas of the body, such as the ovaries, fallopian tubes, bowel and intestine), underscores the assumption that reproductive health issues are related to sexual behavior instead of reproductive issues.

Quinlan and Johnson (2017) suggested that gynecologists didn't believe that Black women could contract endometriosis, which had long been characterized as a "white woman's disease" until 1960. But evidence suggests that African-American women can suffer from higher rates of endometriosis and fibroids.

Biases around diagnosis and treatment
Biases within the medical community exist, and our experiences early on teach us, as people of color, to expect it. While in graduate school, I experienced persistent pelvic pain. During my exam, my gynecologist dismissed my concerns and diagnosed me with PID. After conducting research on my own and enduring several more months of pain, I went back to the doctor. Eventually, an ultrasound revealed two large fibroids (the size of a grapefruit and a lemon) protruding from my uterus.

Years later, when I sought help for fertility issues with therapists and coaches, I didn't feel seen or validated in terms of my racial experience and its impact on my fertility. One practitioner even told me that "Africans are having babies later in life," as a misguided way to soothe my anxious spirit.

With the existence of mistrust for the medical community amongst the African American community around basic medical care, can you imagine what it's like trying to access specialized treatment for infertility?

Representing the black experience

The lack of representation and understanding of racial experiences within the fertility world is another barrier to accessing care. It's easy for people to dismiss the argument of racism when racial issues have never negatively impacted them. When you've seen your story represented everywhere all your life, it can be hard to accept that a person of color experiences it through a different lens.

Being Black in the infertility world means not seeing your story represented in the very communities it's designed to support. It means there's no guarantee you can see a doctor of your own race who'll approach your case with racial sensitivity. It's one of the reasons my communities fight so hard for representation because it matters.

Racial trauma and infertility trauma are interconnected. But for Black women who experience both, the intersection is rarely discussed or even acknowledged in either community.

Dr Loree Johnson @drloreejohnson

Link to the blog: https://drloreejohnson.com/infertility-trauma-is-racial-trauma/

Indians and infertility

Based on the blog post: Me, Myself and IVF

When I was a girl, seeing couples kiss in a film I was watching with my parents was mortifying. It must have been equally embarrassing for them as they'd surreptitiously change the channel to something less risqué, like the news. As soon as I was old enough to predict this scenario, I'd offer to make some tea to escape the awkwardness.

The Bollywood films I watched growing up rarely showed couples kissing. Expressing sensuality was acceptable; sexuality was not. While things are changing, we still struggle to portray sex on-screen or speak about it amongst ourselves. Except ...

There's one aspect of sex that Indians love discussing: making babies. Until you get married, girls are discouraged or even banned from having boyfriends, and you're lucky if you're told about periods, what to expect and how to cope. The moment the ink dries on your marriage certificate, however, mothers, grandmothers and aunties start piling the pressure on to 'get busy beneath the sheets' to continue the family name.

The comments I heard were gentle nudges at first: "It'll be your turn next." Then mildly offensive: "Of course you look glamorous, you don't have kids!" to the wildly inappropriate unsolicited advice: "You should get a move on before your womb shrivels up."

The more insistent they were, the more I distanced myself, doubting whether I wanted children. I have always hated conforming to stereotypes and this was no different. I resented being told what I should be doing with my body and by when. Back then, though, I lacked the courage or vocabulary to express my feelings and fears to my elders, and even if I had, it would have felt disrespectful to disagree with them.

The pivotal moment arrived when I fell pregnant naturally. Instead of the paralysing fear that I'd expected to feel – loss of independence, identity and my figure – I was elated. My expectations couldn't have been further from my real-life feelings; the pressure to procreate had suppressed my interest in motherhood. I envisioned our duo becoming a trio, delighted that the second-hand baby clothes which had been living in our loft would finally be used. Smells were heightened, wine was shunned, and gestures protecting my stomach became reflex actions.

I was still getting my head around this life-changing event and my reaction to it when I was told that I'd miscarried. As the nurse completed the ultrasound scan, I numbly registered that one in four pregnancies in the UK end in miscarriage. I was a stranger to this sad statistic until that day.

We are also a percentage of the one in six British couples who struggle to conceive. After this devastating outcome, we underwent a year of fertility tests and awaited results before being referred for our first IVF (invitro fertilisation) cycle. Seeing all the syringes, needles and medications pushed me over the edge, making me question why we were putting ourselves through this physical and emotional pain.

It amazes me how quickly we adapt when we must. Sinking needles into my skin, popping pills and inserting pessaries became the norm four years ago when we started this cycle. It was unsuccessful, as were the three subsequent cycles, conducted at two different clinics.

While my rational brain knows that infertility is a 'disease of the reproductive system', as defined by WHO, I still feel like a failure. As if I'm defective and that even the best clinics in the country cannot help me.

I also feel like I've failed my husband, our families, and our communities. This sense of shame is what prevents many South Asians from speaking out about their fertility issues. Their inability to conceive can bring immense embarrassment to their loved ones, making them a source of gleeful gossip. And it doesn't matter what the issue is as our patriarchal societies will often blame the woman. It will also be her fault if she only gives birth to daughters; sons are revered in our culture because they carry on the family name, provide for their parents in their golden years, and perform the last rites at their funerals. Daughters mean dowries.

59

Many British Asian families have modernised over time, but some still uphold these traditions and beliefs, making their children's lives very difficult. Thankfully, our families have been supportive from the start, although dealing with their disappointment in addition to our own was challenging. This aspect, along with the fear of judgment, ridicule and rejection may deter individuals and couples from talking about their traumatic experiences with their family and friends.

I decided to go public about our infertility in a blog post on Mother's Day in 2019. Having accidentally discovered the TTC (trying to conceive) community on Instagram and receiving an overwhelming amount of understanding, kindness, and support from strangers, I wanted to give back what I'd gained. Despite having an open dialogue with my family, I still felt incredibly isolated after our miscarriage and first two failed cycles. So, I poured my heart into a post, hoping that my words would resonate with anyone in a similar situation, particularly people from South Asian backgrounds, to make them feel validated and less alone.

Since sharing our story, people frame their questions in a more sensitive manner, eager to learn more about how it feels to undergo IVF and alternate paths to parenthood, including our decision to pursue donor egg IVF (DEIVF). However, after a lifetime of burying their emotions to avoid being perceived as weak, some South Asians struggle to find suitable words in this situation, reaching for platitudes like "Just relax and it'll happen" or "Be positive" to fill the awkward silence. Hearing them makes me want to tear my hair out as they feel dismissive and reductive. Hopefully, the more I discuss our experience, the more barriers I can help to break down so that infertility becomes less stigmatised amongst our communities.

Seetal Savla @savlafaire
   Link to blog post: http://www.savlafaire.com/me-myself-and-ivf/

I'm a single African Mum through double donor conception

I decided to have a family as a single African woman. At nearly forty-eight years old, I thought I could freeze my eggs, only to be informed after speaking to a specialist, that my egg reserve was extremely low and would probably not be of great quality. I decided to do IVF (In-Vitro Fertilisation) using both sperm and egg donor. Of course, I had many thoughts about what people would say, especially being a Nigerian single woman. The cultural way, even today, is that children are raised in a marriage. It's unheard of to be single and trying to start a family alone through double donation. However, I was fortunate that I got pregnant on the frozen embryo transfer and had my baby nine months later.

My journey wasn't easy, but after two failed relationships I decided that I'd had enough tears and anger as to why I was treated badly. And I desperately wanted to have children of my own. My sister has two boys, and my nieces and nephews all had a family of their own. I was smiling on the outside but crying on the inside each time I gave my congratulatory calls.

I buried myself in my work, so I could at least save up for IVF treatment, which cost thousands of pounds. I shopped around till I found a private clinic who would help me and ended up having many tests which were necessary prior to selecting my donor. I was happy that things were moving forward but it was also a costly and lonely project. People don't talk much about the expense of fertility both financially and emotionally. There's no funding for single women who can equally give a loving home to a child. I know because I cried to my General Practitioner, who said I'd have to self-fund my treatment as there isn't any for single women. In the end, I took out a loan to fund my cycle.

The clinic was in Europe and offered me ethnic donated eggs and sperm. I jumped at the chance. After choosing the number of eggs I needed, six embryos where created and one was transferred. I was very excited when I had my transfer, but I couldn't share this news with anyone. The anxiety of waiting for the pregnancy blood test was very tough. When the nurse called me to say that the test was positive, I froze, unable to believe my blessing.

I chose to keep this experience a secret. Why you may ask? Well, what's the alternative? My parents thought I got pregnant from a relationship that went wrong. Thankfully, they've now come round to the situation and are very supportive.

I wrote this for women who want to have a family but are not in a relationship; to let you know that it's possible with the right support from the right clinic. I'm very happy where I am now in my life with my bundle of joy. ANONYMOUS.

Infertile in a fertile country

Infertility has always been just a term to me ... something I learnt in school, something that I wrote down during my exams. It never really registered in my conscious mind, not to talk of couples struggling with infertility – they were scarce in numbers; they were people you remembered and prayed for anytime their name came up in relation to children. I just knew they didn't have kids yet, but I had no idea of the soul-wrenching pain and agony they went through being childless in a society obsessed with children.

Never in my wildest imagination did I think I was going to be twenty-six and still not pregnant. Never did I think that after four-plus years of marriage, I wouldn't have a baby, and instead, have a frustrating diagnosis of 'unexplained infertility'; i.e., no cause could be found. I mean, in my society, the order of things expected is for you to get married and have a baby within the first year of marriage.

Struggling with infertility is hard. Now imagine being infertile in a fertile country, where it seems like couples can have five to ten children just like that. It's doubly hard. Now imagine being unable to have children in a country where being married and having a child is everything; sometimes your respect and status in society depends on it. It's crazy.

Infertility is viewed as a 'woman's thing'; society has been conditioned to think that the woman is the reason why a couple is struggling to conceive, to the extent that religious prayers and even infertility solutions are mostly targeted at the woman. To make matters worse, traditionally, your entire worth as a married woman is tied to supporting your husband and having children. Everywhere, it's the subtle glances, the whispers, the pitying look, or the prayers that put you on the spot, or if you're unlucky, seeing the outright scorn on their faces.

Fertility treatment can be incredibly hard. They don't tell you how it takes a toll on everything – physical and mental health, relationships, life and finances. Every single aspect of your life is affected. Fertility treatment is also incredibly expensive and out of reach for most couples. My hubby and I exhausted all our finances while trying to have a baby and now we can't even afford an IVF cycle. And being unable to have a child naturally has changed me.

Getting support is also hard in a society where things like this aren't discussed in the open. It's all hush-hush. You're not expected to discuss your struggles in public; no one wants to hear about your problems conceiving. It's almost as if it's a thing of shame that needs to be concealed. It makes it incredibly hard, isolating, and lonely.

This is part of the reason I started my Instagram page. It's for women like me to provide support and make the journey a little easier and less lonely for others – a space for us to feel heard in a society that makes us feel less valued for not having children or for only having one child.

Shayo O @naijafertilityhub

It wasn't even a baby yet (miscarriage)

Based on the blog: It wasn't even a baby yet

Six of my seven pregnancies ended in early miscarriage. An early miscarriage happens within the first twelve weeks of pregnancy. But just because it happens within the first three months doesn't make it any less of a loss.

I **hated** it (and still do!) when I hear people's ill-informed and inconsiderate responses to the word miscarriage:
  – "at least it was early"
  – "it wasn't even a baby yet"
  – "it probably didn't even have a heartbeat yet"
  – "at least it didn't happen later on, how much worse would that have been?"
  – "count yourself lucky it happened now".

An early miscarriage is painful and as emotionally heart-breaking as a loss at any other time. Let me explain why ... Imagine wanting something, like *really* wanting it. Let's use an example to make this more relatable. Imagine you want the latest iPhone, you work extra shifts at work, you save a little extra each month, and every other day you find yourself Googling the features to remind yourself of what you'll soon have. You pop into the phone shop just to look at it, excited that it won't be long till you have one of your own. You imagine yourself using it, showing it to your friends, using the new camera, posting the photos from it. You imagine yourself feeling good, feeling proud that you worked so hard for something and you finally got it! You can't wait! You actually can't wait! Can you picture that? Can you feel that excitement?

Now imagine how much deeper the dreams, the excitement, the longing, the anticipation would be if the thing you *really* wanted was a baby, not an iPhone. Can you imagine that? When you see the blue lines on the pregnancy test, possibly after a difficult journey to even get pregnant. Can you imagine the sheer excitement? The feeling that you're on the journey to finally getting what you always wanted; flooded with love, with longing, with connection to the little life that is starting its journey inside you; every day checking your pregnancy app to see how big your baby is and what features are developing; talking to it even though you know it can't hear yet, writing your hopes in your journal, tenderly touching your tummy, wondering if it will be a boy or a girl; your excitement gaining momentum. And you don't know how you'll keep this a secret especially with the beaming smile that you can't seem to remove from your face.

Now imagine that out of the blue, you feel pain, keeled over with cramping, you lose blood, it feels like you're having contractions, you're confused at what's happening; you want to pretend nothing is wrong but you know it is … and at that moment, or days later you finally 'pass' your baby – it's

68

sitting in the bowl of the toilet, and you scream at the thought, mortified that at some point you're going to have to flush the toilet and let what remains of your baby be flushed away in the most undignified manner. Yes, my friends, this is how so many early miscarriages happen ... not in the comfort of a hospital bed like the picture painted in many soap operas.

That life you longed for, the dreams you dreamt, the hopes you had are all gone. You actually feel like your heart has broken in two. You're emotional. The smile you wore has vanished. The excitement has been replaced with a dark cloud. You're finding it all a bit too hard.

And now imagine the sting, the dagger, the sheer cruelty of these words ...
  – 'at least it was early'
  – 'it wasn't even a baby yet'
  – 'it probably didn't even have a heartbeat yet'
  – 'at least it didn't happen later on, how much worse would that have been?'
  – 'count yourself lucky it happened now'.

Do you see how a baby that's longed for and lost, at whatever stage can be a deep and profound loss? Never should that loss be greeted with the inconsiderate and uncompassionate words as depicted above. A loss is a loss no matter when it happens. Use your words wisely.

Gurinder Mann @adrugnamedhope
   Link to the blog https://adrugnamedhope.com/2019/10/09/it-wasnt-even-a-baby-yet/

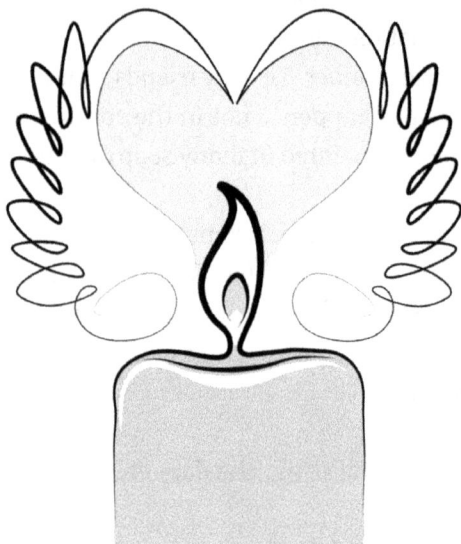

'Wave of Light' to commemorate all babies who sadly died too soon.
(A global event at the end of Baby Loss Awareness Week in October)

The isolation of secondary infertility

"Black people don't have infertility, Kezia! Even women starving in Africa have babies!" she said, in an irritated kinda-way as if I was being naïve about how fertility works. And then she stalked off as if the pep-talk was done. That was said to me by a loving (yes really), relative almost ten years ago, and yet the sting of these words still rings loudly in my ears.

When you go through infertility as a black woman, you experience the isolation of being misunderstood everywhere. Family, friends, media, social media – nowhere is your experience reflected back at you. I remember thinking, *so what does that say about me as a black woman if I can't get pregnant?* What does it mean? What's *wrong* with me? It turned out there was nothing medically wrong with me – in fact, not long after my relative's words, I was pregnant and went on to have a healthy baby boy. What I didn't know then was that I'd struggle to have any more.

Unexplained secondary infertility is defined as the inability to become pregnant or to carry a pregnancy successfully after previous success in delivering a child. So, if the black community isn't talking about primary infertility, then it's certainly not speaking about secondary infertility.

This isn't about whose pain is worse; it's about awareness so that women, especially black women can be supported in a way that's inclusive of a fully lived human experience. That means we can experience fertility issues at any age, at any time and stage in our lives, through no fault of our own.

A part of the problem is the general perception of the 'fertile' black woman and man; since slavery, it's been suggested that black women are naturally fertile, even hyper-fertile. I mean, why else do we look at third world countries perplexed that even in their dire circumstances they're still able to have children. The media does nothing to quash this idea either as we see appeals for all the poor starving black and brown children in remote parts of the world. Except this *is* a stereotype and it's a damaging one.

When you grow up within a community with this belief that 'infertility isn't a thing' and then you find yourself unable to get pregnant or have a second pregnancy after a healthy first-born – you naturally feel immense shame, embarrassment, inadequacy and hopelessness. You become 'othered' again. You carry the feeling of 'other' as a black woman in most areas of life, and society, but then to be othered from your own community, not intentionally, but out of lack of awareness, is hard to bear.

I felt extremely isolated; I had a child and longed for another one. We were happily married, a loving little family. I could tell that people were perplexed as to why, as they wrongly assumed, we had stopped at one. There were so many comments – not just the: "when is the next one coming?" It was the more flippant ones, almost incredulous such as: "you can't have just one!"

What if one child is all I get? I stopped saying 'only' because it made me feel ungrateful for the family I do have. In truth, the "only one?" comments stung too. I knew how hard it was to conceive just one child, so, I felt a growing resentment to those who couldn't understand the struggle to conceive more than one.

The black community certainly takes fertility as a given, and society, in general, doesn't give much thought to fertility until there's a problem with how our bodies are functioning. Sexual health education certainly lacks this basic acknowledgment and works on the presumption that prevention and scaring is better than real knowledge of fertility in both men and women.

But the truth is, it is a problem, albeit a silent one. Did you know that infertility is estimated to affect around twelve per cent of women under the age of forty-four and that black women are twice as likely to struggle as white women? Did you know that only eight per cent of black women will speak to their doctor or seek medical help compared to fifteen per cent of white women?

This is what we're talking about; black women being adversely affected and less likely to speak out about it. Perhaps, we need more safe spaces in which to do so. Perhaps within the anonymity of the internet, social media and Zoom culture, this may happen on a larger and much-needed scale. Because it's not just about accessing treatment, it's about the shared experience, knowing that someone else has been in your shoes or is walking your same path – there is comfort and healing in that. The black community should be a safe haven and it's not; our families should be safe spaces and they're not, because either no one *is* talking about it, doesn't know *how* to talk about it or you are *shamed* for talking about it.

Why? Perhaps because it doesn't fit the narrative of who we're told we are as black people, as black women. It's not a part of our cultural identity. I know that infertility was never spoken about in my family, despite having an aunt who'd never had children and ended up having a hysterectomy in her early forties. In my family, it was a simple divide – those who wanted children and those that didn't. Struggling to have children didn't enter the equation. I'm the first to have experienced it. I'm the first to have brought the conversation to the table. What a difference it would make to have open and honest conversations about the complexities of the childbearing years that we women face.

What I've learnt and what I want black women to know is that infertility is a stumbling block on the way to parenthood, not a pre-determined reality. The more black and ethnic women are educated on fertility and their options, the more knowledge they can use to permeate the culture and instigate conversations. Change is needed. But we need to change the narrative first.

Kezia Ashley Okafor @iamkeziaokafor

Anything goes when you're trying to conceive

Mikvah: is a bath used for the purpose of ritual immersion in Judaism to achieve ritual purity. Today, traditional immersion is usually explained as a spiritual purification, to mark the passing of potential life that comes with each menstrual cycle.

If it happens in the world of infertility, I've been through it. OK - that isn't fair or true, because no two women go through the exact same journey while trying to become a mother. On my harrowing six-year journey to motherhood, I tried EVERYTHING. I mean it - in addition to the extensive ART (Assisted Reproductive Technology), I got to a point where I did *almost* anything someone recommended, because they'd heard it worked for their friend's cousin who now has five kids.

I did the more talked about things: acupuncture, herbs, prayer, Geritol vitamins, squeaky clean eating for a long chunk of time: no gluten, dairy, or processed sugar. (That didn't get me anywhere in terms of pregnancy so I decided that pizza, snickers, and wine felt much more comforting). I also did the less talked about reiki, energy work, intuitive readings, tarot, Epsom salt tricks of all kinds, and eventually, mikvah.

I am a Los Angeles woman so I was obviously doing yoga, too. I befriended my yoga teacher, Julie - nothing fancy, but we'd stand outside the yoga classroom schmoozing until class started to get a glimpse into each other's lives. Julie was a happily single woman well into her thirties, when all of a sudden, she met and married a modern Orthodox Jewish man and had three kids within five years, squeezing it all in just before she turned forty. We connected, Julie and I. She knew when I was getting married, and she knew that several years into my marriage I still didn't have any children (reminder: in that time, she had **three**!). One day after class, Julie put her hands on my belly area and said "So, I have to ask...?" She stared at me with eyes that were trying to go deep into my soul and get answers. My heart sank into my stomach and I looked away, surprised that I didn't just burst into tears right there.

I'd been asked all the questions before: Did we want kids? When did we want kids? How did we want kids? What were we waiting for? And the longer our wait was stretching, the more scared I'd become that someone would ask. We carry so much weight as infertiles. We carry grief, anger, pain, jealousy...being asked the questions about life plans that people assume are natural questions put me into an immediate state of defensiveness, because I was carrying so much pain and anger.

In my heartbroken fuel raged anger and pain, I snapped back at her saying "Thanks for asking. I have tried **everything**...we have done four IUIs and we're about to move onto IVF. I am doing acupuncture, energy work, and praying. Nothing is working, nothing." Without missing a beat, Julie asked "Have you gone to the mikvah?"

I had been to a mikvah once in my life a few nights before my wedding in 2010. Without knowing much about the *why* behind the tradition, I felt it was a special one because as I remembered it, it was an opportunity for a mother-daughter bonding ritual as they went together (as I did with my mother), to usher in a new phase of life. My mother watched me 'dunkin' in accordance with the rules I had been given. We laughed and cried, and had a meaningful experience.

But I had never heard of going to the mikvah as a method for overcoming fertility struggles. I knew it was a way to track ovulation: seven days post end of period you went as an ovulation ritual to go home to your husband cleansed to make a baby. But the way I saw it, if a mikvah couldn't actually impregnate me, what was the point? And yet, in my spinning thoughts of ways to get pregnant, I couldn't get Julie's suggestion out of my head. After all, I consider myself a spiritual person, and Jewish women have been going to mikvah for eons. Of all the crazy things I was doing, I figured I could at least give it a try.

I googled 'Los Angeles Mikvah,' and eventually picked a place that seemed local, clean, and well-reviewed. I called to figure out the logistics and was given the rules; namely no nail polish and seven days post period, and what time to show up. I was nervous to go to the mikvah. Like, irrationally nervous. I was thinking about what I should wear (*do I need to wear a skirt?*), the rules, the asks, the women who may be there judging me knowing that I didn't know the rules. The entire experience is predicated on secrecy. It happens only at night, in my case I entered in the back of a building, down a dark alley. The multiple doors I entered each had a security buzz feature and video surveillance. Why was there so much mystery? I entered, unsure, and self-conscious.

I was greeted with warmth. I was even complimented on my very secular outfit (I went with something that was very me: leggings and a faux fur vest which was a big hit)! I was given a host of instructions: where and how to bathe, the right way to comb my hair to ensure no knots (*obstacles*), a self-care package with q-tips, eye makeup remover... a way to remove any possible obstacles that came between my body and the way God made me. I was shown into a beautiful, private spa-like bathroom, given a plush robe, a pair of slippers, and was told to use the phone inside to call 'o' when ready to take my spiritual dunk. The small spa rooms - there were about ten of them - all had one door in, and one door out to the communal religious experience pool where we'd enter and dunk, one at a time.

I closed the door and looked around this stunning bathroom and realized what an incredible opportunity I'd received. I almost fell down with relief, excitement, understanding. I'd been given a place where I could stop, think, meditate. I was forced to take care of my body, pay attention to what it was doing, telling me. Honestly, it felt like a gift.

Once I fully cleaned myself, pressed 'o' I was escorted into a larger room with the actual mikvah bath. It *almost* reminded me of a bath you'd see on Game of Thrones — it was cavernous, deep into the ground, and it felt very private and very sacred. There was a prayer on the wall in Hebrew and English which I was encouraged to read - I did so with my hand on my heart -

it spoke of family building, and love, and marriage, and I read it slowly and carefully to ensure that whomever was listening to my prayers was really hearing them.

I was checked by the attendant: I disrobed, and she looked at every inch of my body to ensure I was kosher to enter the actual mikvah. Yes, it was strange. I felt weird, and a little awkward and judged. But I also marveled at this woman — a secret woman in the basement of a building in Los Angeles, who shared these moments of quiet prayer with countless women, each of whom came to the mikvah with hope, or maybe grief, excitement, or love.

And I was off. She ushered me down four large stone steps and into the ritual bath. Once in, I dunked three times and read a prayer. She deemed my service kosher, and I re-robed and went back into my spa bathroom through the inside door. It was over so quickly!! SO much build up, preparation, rules, guidelines, panic - and then dunk, dunk, dunk, and out.

But when I entered my bathroom, I felt different. I reflected on the power of water. It is so cleansing, so refreshing. There was a rebirth that happened, a renewal. I felt awakened spiritually in a way I hadn't in a long, long time. After battling to become a mother for so long — after so many slaps in the face, and failed attempts, and doctors, and nurses, and scheduled sex — I needed this awakening more than I realized.

I went back to the mikvah every month that I was trying to get pregnant, and then some months when I wasn't. I went back after my first miscarriage, and eventually my second. I went when I had a terrible fight with my husband. I went when I couldn't think clearly, or was depressed. I went every time I needed a reset. After every failed embryo transfer, every bit of bad news, off I'd go in the night.

Now, I don't know what the rules are for going to the mikvah when you're just in need of some solace, but I found that if it connected me with God in a deeper way, no one would judge me based on the rules. Once I was eventually pregnant with my twins, I even went with another sceptic friend trying for her own IVF miracle. There is a tradition that if a pregnant woman goes and dunks first, and then immediately afterwards the woman who wants to become pregnant dunks, good spiritual mojo will transfer. That was a tradition I could get on board with!

I didn't see Julie for a long while after I became a regular mikvah-goer. But when I did, I nearly cried. She didn't say a word about my unpregnant belly, but I ran to her, hugged her, and told her that she changed my life. I don't credit the mikvah with giving me my twins. But I know for sure that in addition to spiritual growth, I found a loving and peaceful ritual around a time in a woman's life that can be so painful. The peace, the stillness, the cleansing, were all part of my mental health journey through infertility, and remain a solace for me today as a mother.

Abbe Meryl Feder @abbefeder

IVF is nothing to be ashamed of

IVF (In-Vitro Fertilisation) was something that I thought other people went through. Not me. I had a child. She'd been conceived naturally so IVF wasn't something I'd ever considered. Within the community it was always spoken about negatively: "She had a 'test-tube baby' because there was something wrong with her," or "She shouldn't have left it so long, now she can't have children naturally." I never paid much attention, though, because it was nothing to do with me, something I didn't need to know about ... I had a child already, conceived naturally.

I gave birth to my first child in 2007. A few years later we were ready to try for another, only the months turned to years and nothing happened. The GP wasn't very helpful, after all, I'd already had one child so there can't be anything 'wrong with me.'

Then there were the questions... 'Why haven't you had another child?' 'Don't you want another baby?' 'You SHOULD have another baby,' 'Are you trying for another?' 'Don't leave it too long' and so on and on. I dreaded family functions; get-togethers which became opportunities for the aunties to question me, advise me, probe me.

We spent the next five years trying for a baby. Each month was a fresh start. Tracking my basal temperature, using ovulation sticks, sticking to a calendar so we didn't 'miss the window of opportunity,' even on the days when we were tired or stressed. Sixty months of disappointment. Sixty months of not seeing that second line, of taking at least five tests each month, just in case the one before was wrong – then seeing the dreaded red blood which meant that was another month wasted and we'd have to start again. I became consumed with having a baby. I felt envious of others announcing their happy news, having their second, third babies. Don't get me wrong, I was happy for them, but I was sad for me. Why wasn't it me? Then the pang of guilt left me questioning if I was a bad person for feeling envious of others good news.

Five years soon passed. I knew it was time to get a second opinion. To say I was shocked at the diagnosis would be an understatement. PREMATURE OVARIAN FAILURE! (This is when the ovaries stop producing normal amounts of the hormone oestrogen or produce eggs regularly, before the woman is forty years old). My GP failed to pick this up. For years they'd told me there was nothing wrong, my test results were apparently normal, and so it was 'secondary infertility' and nothing they could do about it. I had a child already and I just needed to 'try harder!'

I was now that person, having to decide to undertake the IVF route. Would I be spoken about like I'd heard others being spoken about? I decided to only tell a few people and we started our journey. I was so naïve. I didn't have a clue about how I'd feel, what it would entail, how time-consuming IVF was, how meticulous I'd have to be with medication timings, how many appointments I'd have to attend. I just did what I was told by the consultant and put my total faith in her and the process. The injections were hard. They hurt. The worst one was the progesterone injection that went into my butt. My husband would have to inject this one as I couldn't reach around. My heart rate would be racing for several minutes afterwards. I found the Clexane one easiest as it was in my stomach and I could inject it myself. It was easier as it was spring-loaded, and by the end of the cycle, I became a pro at injecting myself.

Unfortunately, the first cycle ended in a chemical pregnancy (early miscarriage). I was devastated. I'd never heard of chemical pregnancies and the consultant hadn't mentioned this as a possibility. To make it worse, a few people I'd confided in didn't seem to understand. One told me that I should just adopt as there were plenty of girl children in India that people didn't want, and another told me that I should be grateful as I had one child already.

I was adamant that I wouldn't go for a second IVF cycle. I didn't want to go through all of that again and have nothing at the end. However, the consultant persuaded me to try again. She said the fact that I'd got pregnant, despite it ending in a chemical pregnancy, was a good sign and that I should give it another chance. I reluctantly agreed. At least this time, I knew what to expect. I decided not to tell anyone else this time, except for two of my closest colleagues. They were my rocks throughout, especially as I hadn't told my employers, which was difficult as I was attending so many appointments. Unfortunately, this cycle also didn't work.

I felt deflated and upset; the thought of having to undergo the whole process again was daunting. At the same time, I felt stronger and more informed. I'd done a lot of research and was a lot more confident. I knew exactly what questions to ask, what I could and should expect from the clinic and the consultant, what was available to me, and that I had the right to change clinics ... which I did. I'd lost faith in the clinic I was using; something didn't feel right, especially after I'd asked about a new protocol I'd researched or had a question about why my cycles so far hadn't worked – the response was very much that they were the professionals and knew what they were doing, which didn't answer my questions. I felt a lot more confident at this stage simply because I was more informed.

I found a clinic in Cyprus and contacted them. Before I knew it, I was preparing for the third cycle. This clinic had so many options available, from an embryoscope, (the embryos are monitored by time-lapse photos so they don't have to be removed from the incubator), to pre-genetic testing (a cell is removed from the embryo and tested for genetic problems). I asked for everything to be included just so I could say, 'I gave it my best shot.' At this stage, I was prepared for this to be our last attempt and wanted to feel like I'd given it my all. However, thinking back I'm sure had this cycle not worked, I would have carried on trying. The thought of looking back and thinking 'what if' would have driven me mad.

The two-week wait was torture. As always, I analysed every

single twinge, feeling, and pregnancy sign. I wanted to feel confident that it would be positive, but I didn't want to get my hopes up for another disappointment. I wanted to carry on as normal but I couldn't think of anything else. The two-weeks that feels like two years!

The day of the test finally came around and I'd promised myself that I wouldn't use a stick test, but instead, wait for the clinic to get back with the hCG test (a blood test which checks for the pregnancy hormone) – that was a long day! The phone didn't ring until gone 5 p.m. – the test was POSITIVE. IT WORKED! I was still afraid though, that it would be taken away from me like with the first cycle. That test had been positive too, only to then turn into a negative. I remained cautious. I must have done at least five tests a day until my six-week scan, then another five a day until my twelve-week scan! I then booked a private scan at every opportunity just to put my mind at rest. It wasn't until I was quite far along into the pregnancy that I allowed myself to relax, but I never totally relaxed until I had my baby in my arms.

For a while, I didn't tell anyone that I'd undergone IVF as I didn't want the stigma attached that's so prevalent in Indian communities. I didn't want anyone pointing fingers at me and saying there was something wrong or blaming my lifestyle, or that I'd left it until my thirties to start a family. I didn't want people pointing at my child and calling her the 'test-tube baby.'

But then, I changed my mind. WHY? Why should I keep quiet? I'd undergone an amazing journey to complete my family – a rollercoaster of a journey – one that wasn't easy by any means.

I'd taken medication orally and internally, injected myself daily, had umpteen scans, was poked, prodded, and had three smear tests when I was used to putting them off for as long as possible! How could I keep this to myself? How many other women were going through this alone? Afraid of being stigmatised. No-one to talk to, making up excuses to attend appointments, to leave the room to administer yet another injection, to smile through the two-week wait when your insides felt all knotted as you prayed for a positive test result ... just so you didn't have to go through all of it again. Why should I keep quiet when I'd undergone something so special, something that came with no guarantees, but I went ahead regardless?

I talk about my journey openly on social media and I've had so many women message me to thank me for sharing my journey, because it gave them the courage to seek professional help; something they'd put off because of the stigma around IVF in the Indian community. Some women still aren't confident enough to tell their families but are grateful they're not alone. Women who've opened up because they've realised that there's nothing to be ashamed of, but everything to be proud of, and those that just want advice.

If we don't share our journeys, we can't help anyone. IVF is nothing to be ashamed of. I look at my family every day with gratitude. We are blessed, we made this happen. We completed our family. What's shameful about that?

Manjeet Sahota @fitspiration_fitter

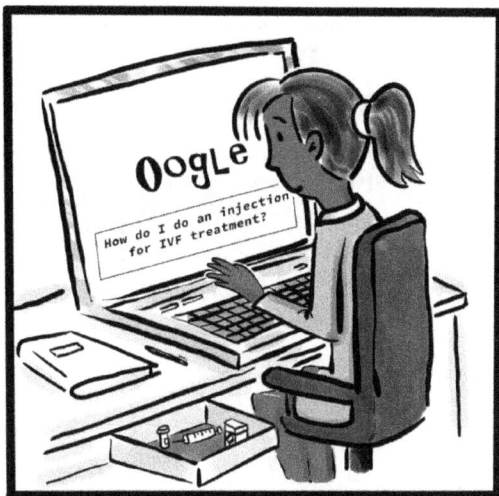

Doing IVF when working – most people
have chocolate in their desk drawer...

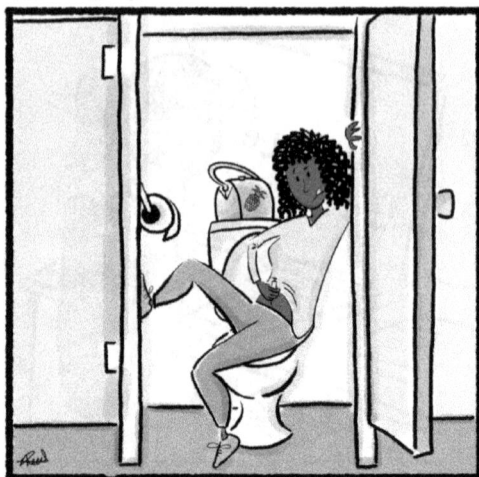

Sometimes you have no choice where you do the
injections – today, the toilet at work…

The truth about IVF

Infertility is a medical condition and unlike other illnesses usually affects two people.

IVF is a medical procedure as it involves medications, injections, blood tests, scans, surgery and a myriad of emotions. Let me explain:

- Consultations with a doctor, sometimes several
- Blood tests to measure hormone levels – lots of and regularly
- Scans of your ovaries and your womb lining
- Losing your dignity from said scans
- Often minor, sometimes major surgery for endometriosis, fibroids, scar tissue
- The man masturbating and not for pleasure, to produce sperm samples
- Sniffing a nasal spray
- Injections – hundreds, possibly thousands of them if over several cycles
- Bruises from the injections
- Side effects from the medications – bloating, headaches, nausea, mood swings

- Surgery to hopefully collect eggs – it's not always successful
- Hours spent on researching everything about fertility treatments
- A massive financial bill for most people that causes additional stress
- Years of tears, anger, sadness, depression, worry, sleepless nights, pain, hurt, hate, envy, lost friendships
- Takes away the spontaneity in your sex life and your life
- A baby is not going to be created through making love but through science
- It's not two people making a baby, instead there's a team:
- - Doctors
- - Nurses
- - Embryologists
- - Sonographers
- - Pharmacists
- - Egg donor (maybe)
- - Sperm donor (maybe)
- - Embryo donor (maybe)
- - Clinic receptionists
- - Counsellor
- - Coach (maybe)
- - Acupuncturist (maybe)
- - Nutritionist (maybe)
- - Reflexologist and other holistic practitioners (maybe)
- - Bank manager (possibly) to pay for this team, and all the home ovulation and pregnancy tests
- - A community of others cheering you on and watching you back – priceless
- It takes over your life; it creeps into every area until you

can't remember what your life was like pre–IVF
- It's not guaranteed to be successful. Let me say that again; it's not guaranteed
- A lot of patience is needed for all the waiting
- There's no excitement in missing a period and wondering...
- Not being able to surprise your partner with a positive pregnancy test because you both know when test day is
- It makes you extremely anxious when you get a positive pregnancy result.

Sheila Lamb @fertilitybooks

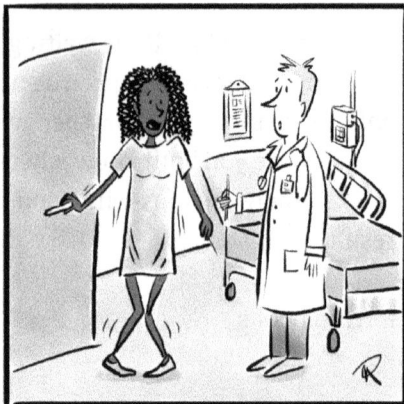

"Now, you absolutely promise
me it won't fall out?"

Sharing is caring (infertility)

*A chapter from the book: **Semen Secrets***

Semen Secret: You are the only one who is dealing with infertility. No one else knows how you feel. No one knows what it's like to be denied something you want so bad.

Conversations about kids with my friends had become awkward. The few who knew about our issue would try to be super polite. I appreciated the gesture, but it did not negate the fact that I wanted what they had. When people complained about their children or about being pregnant, I would get so angry. To complain about the very thing I wanted so desperately, seemed horribly inconsiderate. Sometimes I felt that they took having a baby for granted. I wanted to remind them, *be thankful because everyone can't have a baby*. The nasty tones would often slip out before I could put them back in my mouth. My friends would follow with, "I'm sorry girl, that's not what I meant. Did I offend you?" Their apologies were genuine, but the damage had already been done. I was reminded that I still lacked what I wanted most.

I would try not to roll my eyes as I smiled back and insisted it was okay. Sometimes I was the one who had to apologize when I imposed my feelings on them. My pain was my own to bear. I was alone in my world. Alone in my thoughts. I had yet to meet anyone who understood what it was like to go through what I was going through.

I hated when people with kids would try to sympathize. "I know how you feel," they would say, "I have kids, but it was still a struggle." They had no clue how I felt. They couldn't know. And I was tired of hearing, "Just stay strong." It was bullshit. "Maybe God has a different plan." What plan was that? Did his plan include giving us back the time we had already lost? Everyone tried to make me feel better, but what no one understood was that there was no feeling better. I believed my situation was an anomaly—there was no one on this earth who could empathize with me or guide me or fix it, let alone make me feel better about it.

For years I had ridden an emotional roller coaster. I would go from ranting to simmering in my feelings. I would look through social media posts from my friends and see other people's baby reveals, birth announcements, bulging bellies, and adorable babies. Then I would cry, get angry, smile, be jealous, get depressed, or curse the computer only to open it back up to look at more pictures.

One day I opened my Facebook page to begin my ritual of drowning in my sorrows and saw that one of my sorority sisters was announcing her baby. *But when was she pregnant?* She had a social at her house not too long ago, she didn't talk about her baby. Did I miss something?

The next day I mentioned to my husband that she had a baby, "I think she adopted it." I thought I was against adoption; the process was brutal and it came with risks. What if the child had emotional issues? What if the kid had genetic defects and got sick? What if the adopted parents changed their mind and wanted the child back? What if the child wanted to find their real parents and left me and my husband? Adoption was terrifying the more I thought about it. Plus, I wanted to be pregnant, experience those labor pains everyone was complaining about, and most of all, hold a child in my arms who reflected me and my husband's characteristics.

But, did I want to be pregnant more than I wanted to raise a child, more than I wanted someone to call me mommy and him daddy? Month after month, my priorities changed and after seeing the Facebook post I decided that I didn't just want to be pregnant, I really wanted to have a baby. When I mentioned the post to my husband, he suggested I reach out to my sorority sister. I was shocked that he would encourage me to share our story with someone and look into adoption again, maybe his priorities were changing too.

I was nervous about calling her. We weren't close friends and we had never had a conversation more intimate than, "How are you?" I almost didn't reach out to her but then, as chance would have it, I saw her at a sorority meeting and I mustered up the courage to ask her if I could give her a call.

She said, "Sure," and that was that. On the way home, I rehearsed how I was going to ask her about her baby: *I didn't know you were pregnant.* Too obvious, because clearly, she

95

wasn't pregnant. *So, where did you get your baby?* It sounded like I was asking her where she brought her shoes. More worrisome than how I was gonna ask her about her baby, was how I'm going to tell her about my situation. Did I really want a near-stranger to know my husband's sperm didn't exist? What would she think about him? Maybe she was someone who would understand what I was going through. Maybe if I knew her situation my anxiety would go away. Which meant, I had to make the call.

What was the use of hiding behind the rawness of the pain of wanting a child when there was someone who may be able to help me get through it all? I took a deep breath and dialed her number. I was hoping she wouldn't answer, but on the third ring, I was forced to face my fear. "Hey lady," she answered.

"Hi," I muttered, unsure of myself.

"So, what did you want to talk about?"

It's funny how you rehearse things in your head and then, when it's time to have the conversation, you just spill your guts in earnest. "Well...umm...I wanted to ask you about your recent Facebook post. I haven't told anyone this, and I'm not sure why I'm telling you, but my husband and I have been unable to have a baby, and I told him I saw you with a baby that I think you adopted. So, he told me I should call you and find out. But you can tell me if I'm too much in your business. I'll understand."

She burst into laughter. I was trying to figure out what I said that was so funny. "In my business? Please, I put it on Facebook. Yes, my husband and I adopted a baby girl. I always wanted a baby and after $60,000 and two failed IVF treatments, I finally have a baby girl."

I inhaled sharply, "$60,000? That is a lot of money."

"Yes, it is," she agreed. "But, when I got this baby, it was all worth it. It wasn't easy though. I've been through hell to get here. Lost my mind chile."

"I'm losing my mind too," I admitted, breathing a sigh of relief. "I torture myself with questions about why God is holding up the process. Sometimes, I try to convince myself that the delay is just giving us time to build up our finances, learn our family history, take more trips. Maybe God has a sense of humor or he is just testing my faith."

I paused, not sure I was ready to share more details, but then I didn't want to lose this opportunity to confide in someone who might finally understand. I took a deep breath and shared that my husband had no sperm. "I always resolve that at the next doctor's appointment God will finally release the sperm and make us parents. But I'm still waiting." My voice got a little louder as I continued, "I'm sick of people telling me to pray. Pray? I'm angry at God. Yes, angry. All women are supposed to have babies and even though they say God doesn't make bad things happen to you, the devil had to get permission from him to do so right? So that means that God saw this coming, and he didn't stop it."

I was panting, angry and feeling fully justified in my anger. She identified with the pain, the fear, the anger, the grief, even the small wins and, of course, the major defeats. She knew my story. She couldn't identify with her husband having no sperm, but she understood wanting a baby and not being able to get pregnant. Everyone else I talked to had a baby naturally. She was the first person I could talk to who could validate everything I was going through—everything I was feeling. She had gone through IVF and it did not result in a pregnancy. It was similar to my husband going through the testicular biopsy and it not resulting in any sperm. She understood what it was like for people to constantly ask when she was going to have a baby, to decline baby shower invites, to have to get over the fact that the journey to parenthood came at a cost—financially and emotionally. She understood how infertility brought turmoil in the marriage. It felt like the weight that had been pressing on my chest had been lifted.

She joked, "Girl, I have been there and done that, brought a T-shirt, socks, and the mug! It's funny I can laugh about it now but there was a time I would cry all day. So, I'm telling you it will get better, trust that."

It's one thing for my friends and family to tell me that *it's going to be okay*, but it's completely different coming from someone who knows what it feels like when it's not okay. She continued, "I may be forty, but I got my baby! It seems unfair, I know. This should be free. The doctors should be able to fix it all. But, if I didn't go through what I did, I wouldn't be here today trying to keep you from falling off the cliff."

Falling off the cliff? I felt like I had jumped, landed with a sickening thud, and jumped again—several times. I kept coming back to the cliff. I'm not sure where determination left off and insanity took over.

"You can call me anytime," she offered. "Day or night, when-ever the pain hits you. Whenever you're confused, call me and we can talk it through."

From then on, she was my lifeline. Every question I had about adoption, every time someone was insensitive, every time I felt empty or alone, I could call her, and she would always answer... always.

CONFESSION: This is nothing new under the sun. There is always someone who has gone through what you have been through or those who have gone through something worse. I was not an anomaly. There was someone who knew how I felt. However, if she had never shared her story, I would have never found my comforter and confidant. I found that sharing a painful story is caring about others who may be in the same place and need to know they are not alone. I found that God will place the right people in your life when you need them the most, and often, it's a person you least expect. It was the unexpected that met my expectations. Our stories were slightly different but our pain was similar.

TJ Peyten, @tjpeyten

Imagine if... (infertility, IVF, miscarriage & loss)

You'll have to inject yourself daily and you're scared of needles

You'll have to have tests, investigations, painful procedures, scans, blood tests, injections, operations, maybe all for nothing

You're asked multiple times, over many years, "when are you having a baby?"

You're told to 'just relax' over and over again for something that's out of your control

You're always waiting

You've spent all your savings and still there's no baby

You'll never make an announcement on social media that you're pregnant

You'll never be able to say to your partner "I'm pregnant!"

You'll never touch your pregnant belly

You'll never feel your baby move inside you

You'll never attend your own baby shower

You'll never announce the birth of your baby

You'll never hear your baby's first cry

You'll never give your baby their first cuddle

You'll never give your baby a kiss goodnight

You'll never see your baby's first smile or hear them coo

You'll never take your baby's photo with the weekly/monthly

milestone board

You'll never feel the warmth or weight of your baby lying on your chest

You'll never hear your baby say "Mamma" or "Dadda"

You'll never bake and decorate your child's birthday cakes

You'll never sing your favourite nursery rhyme to or with your child

You'll never push your baby on the swing

You'll never make your parents grandparents

You'll never hear your child tell you they love you

You'll never hold your child's hand as you walk down the street together

You'll never jump in muddy puddles with your child or fly a kite

You'll never take them to their first day of school

You'll never hear them read their favourite book to you

You'll never have the memories of your religious or cultural ceremony for your baby or child.

Imagine if you didn't have any memories of these precious moments of pregnancy or of your baby, child or children. Imagine what it's like for us, so desperate to experience all that you have, but not knowing if we'll ever make these memories.

Sheila Lamb @fertilitybooks

The silent sufferer (infertility)

My husband and I were married for two years before we sought the help of a reproductive endocrinologist. My desire to have a child quickly became an obsession. At the time of the first treatment in 2012, I was twenty-nine years old, and the IUI (intra-uterine insemination) cycle was unsuccessful. An x-ray test concluded fallopian tube blockage on the right side. We'd never fallen pregnant on our own, and I'd never previously been pregnant.

We buried ourselves in our work and didn't seek further help until four years later in 2016. Married for approximately five and a half years, I knew there had to be an explanation. Why was my body failing me? My menstrual cycles were regular every month, and nothing appeared to be out of the ordinary. I thought that we'd done everything right. We dated for twenty-three months before marriage. He had a house for us to call home and we were financially stable. Did we not deserve the gift of parenthood? Had we not proven ourselves worthy? I felt grieved at the thought of getting help for the one thing my body should do naturally and with ease. Eventually, I was diagnosed with hypothyroidism and underwent surgery to remove uterine polyps.

I felt isolated for four years trying to find community and support outside of my marriage. Being a silent sufferer gave me a sense of control. I couldn't command my diagnosis to disappear, but I could manage who I shared it with.

Things were a little different at this time and advocacy for infertility was deeply lacking on social media platforms. I scrolled various hash-tags endlessly on Instagram for women with the same circumstances to ease the pain. It was obvious brown women didn't openly express their fertility issues as widely as our Caucasian counterparts. Black and brown women are often perceived as hyper-fertile, a bias, I too, believed. Although both of my grandmothers experienced early miscarriages, they gave birth to eleven children between them. So, what reasons would I have to doubt my ability to conceive naturally? Every family takes note of the common medical conditions that plague them, but no one saw infertility coming.

The emotional turmoil that infertility brings is similar to the waves of the ocean. There are times of high tides and moments of absolute stillness.

I often felt like I should have been warned about infertility. Instead, movies, television shows, and the media portrayed images of the perfect family that included children. No warning of the one in eight couples in the USA diagnosed with infertility.

Becoming an advocate for infertility is probably not your concern and that's okay. It's not the path for everyone. What matters is that you find your voice by connecting with others who understand your situation. Your path to parenthood may not be the typical story represented in the media, but it is yours, and only you can decide how to navigate it.

Monique @infertilityandmepodcast

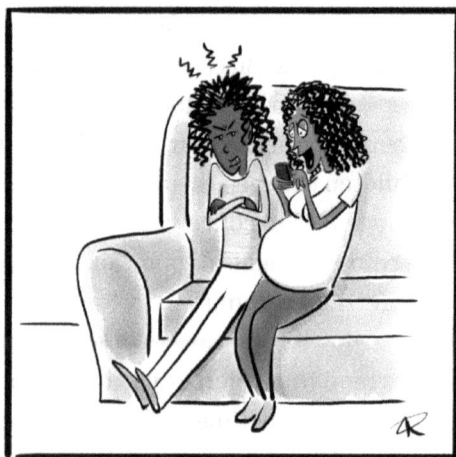

"Try this app, I used it and got pregnant within a month of downloading it!"

And I surrender... (infertility & IVF)

When we got the confirmation that IVF (In-Vitro Fertilisation) would be our only option, I took a mental and emotional break from all things to do with 'trying-to-conceive.' It gave me a renewed perspective about how much light we do or don't let into our lives at times, because we can be tunnel-visioned towards one desire. Making room for other parts of my life, for the multi-dimensional being that I am, made me feel whole again, functional, instrumental in the construction of who I was trying to be and the life I was trying to lead. I've been able to make time for joy, too, meeting and reconnecting with friends and family and occupying spaces that remind me of who I am.

When we first began our investigations, I was very keen on knowing everything. I googled a lot; I read and watched everything I could find, but none of it ever made me feel at ease. What pacified my anxiety was attending each of our appointments and finding out more about our fertility health. The KNOWING, that real concrete knowing about our situation specifically, put me more and more at ease with each appointment.

What you find on Google is often generalised, and what you find on Instagram is often unique to that individual or couple. If your own fertility issues don't apply to either, you can often be left feeling more in the dark as if something is wrong with you. And so now, I've finally come into a space of surrender. To the truth. Our truth. Not speculation. Not generalised information.

When I went to my first appointment at the fertility clinic, I went alone. It was just a blood test, so I figured I'd be fine. But when I got there, I was overwhelmed with so much emotion – the other people in the waiting room were all couples, and I started welling up, but before things got out of hand, I was called in by the nurse. She was matter-of-fact about everything – because, after all, it was just a blood test, and I left after five minutes thinking what was all that emotion about? Our minds can trick us into emotion, but we can also use our minds to control how we feel, and now two failed embryo transfers later, I've been trying to practice this.

I've been thinking a lot about when I'll eventually fall pregnant and have a baby, as a baby is not guaranteed, and I keep imagining myself holding them and looking back at how she or he came about. I'd hate for the memory to be that of pain and sorrow.

I allowed my desire to become a mother to consume a huge part of my life, putting a lot of things on hold because I was always planning for motherhood. I don't subscribe to that way of living anymore, and instead, I want to be like water; occupying spaces that welcome me and swiftly moving past ones that don't. I want my children to be conceived from a place of balance, a place of intention, the right energies, and a place of faith.

The IVF process is a process of scheduling; everything is dictated and controlled to the T. So, my mind has been centred on how I can recreate the bliss of spontaneous (natural) conception in this simulated and very unnatural process. When you go through IVF you know too much, because everything is scheduled and seems so precise and fool-proof (which it really isn't – there's a thirty per cent success rate for under thirty-fives), so it can be very hard to deal with when it doesn't work out.

But surrendering the outcome helps me accept any eventuality with grace. Surrendering doesn't mean I'm giving up hope, not at all ... for me, it simply means, I'm giving up dictating the outcomes and timeframes around our fertility journey, and just giving it all up to God, to science, and intention. We have a true desire to be parents and I believe God will meet that desire, and science will facilitate our preferred outcome.

While my desire for a baby is real and strong, I also desire to be happy with what I have, as I am.

As we approach our four-year mark of trying to conceive, in the words of Danielle Doby, the author of a poetry book called *I Am Her Tribe:*

"I surrender. To the soft. And the sweet. And the sorrow. Not shying away. Allowing each inhale and exhale to source a new life into my cells from their exchange. Within each release, lives an offering. What we let go of creates room for beginnings ... Your winter may last for days, months, lifetimes. But do not mistake this as a dead bloom. Forever closed off to others. For this season isn't for rising, just yet. This season is for letting the light pour itself into our emptied hands."

Noni Martins @unfertility

Healing and wisdom after losing my babies

I found out I was pregnant for the first time shortly before my 31st birthday. It was completely unplanned. My husband and I weren't married at the time or living together. I was enjoying a somewhat nomadic existence working in Manhattan as a swim-wear designer, crashing at my cousin's place in Brooklyn during the week, and then living in Philly on the weekends. I wasn't making much money, so having a child wasn't on my list of priorities. Once I processed the shock of being pregnant, I was overcome with excitement. All of a sudden, I was so in love with this little life growing inside of me that I made all kinds of plans in those first couple of weeks! Thoughts of my baby shower, thinking of names, how I'd give birth, setting up my maternity leave, considering providers for prenatal care, etc.

However, I had spotting throughout my first few weeks. I raised my concerns about it with my OB/GYN but she downplayed it as a common occurrence. By the time I'd reached my eleventh week of pregnancy, the spotting was worse and accompanied by cramping. By the end of that week, I spontaneously mis-carried my first child who I named Carter Gray. I was utterly traumatized by the feeling of my water breaking and seeing my lifeless baby fall from my body. Following the miscarriage, I had excruciating waves of pain and days of heavy bleeding, passing blood clots the size of grapefruits. It wasn't until after I lost Carter that my GYN even mentioned the reality of miscarriage. I was blown away that she'd been so neglectful in conveying how common it was, especially after she was aware that I was showing early signs. I was devastated. I'd never been in so much emotional pain.

A little over a year later, I became pregnant again. I tried my best to manage my stress through this pregnancy. I had early spotting again which sent my anxiety through the roof. Then the spotting subsided and I'd got safely through my first trimester, thinking I was in the clear and feeling more optimistic about my pregnancy. At our scan, I found out I was having a boy and he was growing beautifully. One day, during my nineteenth week, I felt mild waves of pressure in my abdomen. I tried not to overreact and convinced myself that the sensations were normal pregnancy growing pains. Later that evening I felt a gush of blood, which of course sent my husband and I running to the Emergency Room (ER).

I spent hours in the ER before seeing a doctor and then had an ultrasound which revealed that my cervix was funnelling open. The OB who finally came down from the Labor and Delivery (L&D) department to consult with me was a black woman. I was relieved upon seeing her face, thinking that she'd truly help me and my baby in any way possible. To my deep disappointment, she gave me a cold and swift diagnosis of having an incompetent cervix, (where your cervix starts to shorten and open early in the pregnancy), and followed that by saying there was nothing she could do to stop another inevitable miscarriage. Without allowing me any space to think, the OB instructed me to bear down, forcing my water to break. I'll never forget the sense of terror that spread through my body, frozen in a nightmare of losing another child. Very quickly after my water broke, the same OB forced a Cervidil suppository (medication to prepare the cervix for birth), into my cervix without warning or gaining my consent. Her words of advice to me were to try for another baby and then instructed the ER staff to give me whatever I wanted for pain. She also insisted that I be left in the ER instead of being transferred to the L&D department because I wasn't twenty weeks pregnant yet. I was nineteen weeks! In her view, that wasn't far enough along for me to be cared for by experienced L&D nurses and staff. After spending the night in the ER, laboring on my own with my husband, I was finally able to advocate enough to be moved up to L&D. I eventually gave birth to my son, Stokely. He was born sleeping.

I conceived again only five months later. This time, I'd done a bunch of research on doctors that specialized in cervical issues and narrowed down the providers that I felt could give me the best care. I was as vigilant as I could be, asking all kinds of questions and immersing myself in whatever research I could find about pregnancy loss and prevention. I had a cerclage (a stitch placed in the cervix to stop it opening too soon), around my eleventh week of pregnancy by a reputable physician in South Jersey. I continued my care with an MFM (Maternal-Fetal Medicine specialist) practice that I trusted to keep a close eye on me throughout my pregnancy.

After the first genetic screening, I learned that I had a low PAPP-

A (Pregnancy Associated Plasma Protein) reading which was associated with developing pre-eclampsia later in pregnancy. I was already scheduled for bi-weekly ultrasounds starting around twenty-four weeks. I walked on eggshells during my second trimester, praying every day to make it to that all important date where the baby had a good chance of survival.

Thankfully, I passed my twenty-fourth week and felt a bit more optimistic ... that I would finally bring home a living child. At my twenty-eight-week appointment, I learned some disturbing news. One of my doctors reviewed my ultrasound scan and found that my son's umbilical cord was hypo-coiled - meaning the vein and two arteries are less coiled than usual. The doctor recommended that I start coming in for weekly scans to check the baby's heart rate and growth. I didn't know what to think or how to feel. I was in denial that this could result in me losing another child.

A few days after my appointment, I noticed decreased movement. Something felt wrong. After experiencing this for a few hours, I became extremely worried and decided to go to the local hospital and demand an ultrasound. When my husband and I arrived, we frantically told the staff of my previous history and that we just needed to hear a heartbeat. The L&D nurses felt our palpable anxiety and found an old ultrasound machine to check for a heartbeat. I'd seen so many scans before, so I could clearly see ... there was no heartbeat.

I was induced the following day and gave birth to my baby boy, Ellison, also born sleeping.

I felt so lost after losing my third child. This time, I knew I needed to find support for myself outside of my family and friends. I realized that while they were loving and truly had my back, they also had limitations. I also know the vicarious trauma that they experienced via my experience was also something that needed healing; constantly leaning on them would have been unfair. I was carrying a very heavy load. This time, I decided to find a therapist who specialized in pregnancy loss and anxiety. I did video journaling, meditation and aromatherapy before going to bed, as well as lots of praying for peace and strength for myself and my husband. I also found a deep sense of comfort in attending a support group for pregnancy loss that I still attend to this day. Devouring all I could learn about fertility and reproduction also led me to a passion for birth work and thoughts of becoming a doula. I thought about what I wished I'd had, and how I could support families who'd struggled in ways similar to myself.

The day I found out I was pregnant with my daughter Memphys, was the same day of an annual memorial service I attended with the bereaved parent's community in N.Y. I didn't know if this pregnancy would be any different, and if I'd ever bring her home alive, but I felt blessed again with the miracle of life inside of me. I vowed that I'd try like hell not to relinquish my joy to anxiety.

This time, I felt super confident in my MFM provider. She cared for me during the loss of Ellison, so I knew I was in trusted, loving hands. She was super available for me and put all the other doctors in the practice on high alert of the type of attention I'd need. She was compassionate, thorough, and thoughtful, and that was priceless. Aside from staggering morning sickness and a repeat cerclage surgery, my pregnancy with my daughter was healthy and uneventful. To be on the safe side, I decided to have an elected induction at thirty-nine weeks.

The day I went to the hospital for the induction was pretty peaceful and I felt a sense of calm. I took a lot of comfort in knowing that I'd finally be giving birth on my terms. While in labor, I had my eyes peeled to the monitors, watching my little girl's heart rate. I just wanted it to be over as quickly as possible. All I could think was the sooner she was out, the safer she'd be. After laboring for about nine hours, I gave birth to a healthy baby girl we named Memphys. She announced herself with a loud yell at 11:30 a.m. on June 28th, 2019.

I often reflect on everything I've endured during my journey of being a mother and how it's shaped parts of my existence. I'll never forget the pain, but also the love and beauty that I've grown to know intimately through my experiences. I also think about the trauma and grief – how you can be defined by it or grow from it, and I'm grateful for the lessons I learnt about myself through my pain. My spirit is more open and I carry a wisdom and foresight that I didn't have before.

I wish the children that I've lost were with me. There isn't a day that goes by where my heart doesn't ache from knowing they're not here, but their existence, no matter how brief, were miracles. It's so important to highlight the stories that don't have a neatly packaged ending.

So many families suffer in silence when they have a loss. Black families especially often face a lack of support, which is also compounded by neglectful care from the entire healthcare system. These disparities have devastating effects on communities. Being a victim of this covert form of racism was the catalyst for me to become a doula. Doulas are especially needed to advocate for families since the greater community has fallen short. We're here to help bridge those gaps, equipped with knowledge and resources for families to be supported through whatever they're experiencing. We hold space for the hard conversations and tough emotions.

Knowing what it's like to lose a child during pregnancy and having access to resources that can help facilitate a healing environment is a privilege that I am beyond grateful to have. I'm hoping I can pay it forward to as many people who are in need of that compassion and empathy.

Marise Angibeau-Gray @4memphys

I concentrated on feeling good and being in a good headspace (IVF)

I was diagnosed with stage 4 endometriosis in 2012, so when my husband and I decided it was time to start a family, my doctor advised me to go directly for IVF instead of wasting time trying to conceive naturally. For those of you who don't know what IVF is, it's short for In Virto Fertilization. They basically take mature eggs from the ovaries and mix them with the sperm in the hope the eggs are fertilized. Or the sperm is injected directly into the eggs in a similar process called ICSI; Intracytoplasmic Injection. If you're someone with fertility issues, endometriosis, PCOS (Polycystic Ovarian Syndrome), or are just unable to get pregnant, IVF is usually the recommended route. Once the eggs are fertilized and embryos are formed, they put them back into the womb and whether it sticks or not is, of course, up to God.

My husband and I started our journey with IVF in Karachi. Honestly, it was the most traumatizing experience of my life, although, I did everything I could to make myself believe it wasn't a big deal. My husband couldn't be with me throughout, because he couldn't take much time off of work, but luckily, I had my family around.

The thing with IVF is that it feels like your body has been taken over by the worst and most vulnerable side of you. You're injected with two different hormones every day for ten to fourteen days, and then another trigger shot before they go in to remove the eggs. They put you under general anesthesia and use a needle to remove the eggs, which are then fertilized and monitored for up to seven days. For most people, the embryos are transferred back anywhere between five to six days after fertilization, but the entire IVF process revolves around your period cycle. Once the embryos are transferred, you're put on three different hormones to help the embryos take root.

Unfortunately, the stress from all the hormones and the IVF process can take a toll on you physically and emotionally, no matter how strong you are. And boy did it take a toll on me! IVF turns you into a ball of hormones – everyone and everything upsets you and makes you angry. You don't feel like yourself, you don't want to talk to anyone, and when you do talk to someone you end up fighting, snapping, crying, or you spend your entire time trying to stop yourself from fighting, snapping or crying. The hormones can cause severe bloating and weight gain – which it did for me every single time. I felt like I had so much water under my skin that it would rip apart any minute. By the time the bloating went down (which by the way takes forever), it was time to go through it all again.

My husband and I spent four years going through IVF. This meant that any plans I had for my career or my life took a backseat. Everything revolved around 'the next IVF cycle'. I was constantly traveling for my IVF's – first to Pakistan and then to Singapore. I was obsessively dieting, trying to get rid of the bloating and weight gain, and constantly frustrated because it was so hard to drop the weight – and sadly everyone around me constantly reminded me how much weight I'd gained, which was the last thing I needed.

I'm a very strong person. I can handle a lot, but this series of IVFs broke me. I cried uncontrollably every time I got a negative result, but no one around me saw that, including my husband. I was always very open about my IVFs with everyone, but I never talked about what I was going through inside, which I now realize was a mistake. But honestly, you can feel like no one will understand what you're going through, not even your partner, and to be honest, I never really understood what I was feeling.

Yes, your partner is going through it too, but you're the one whose body is taken over by hormones and being poked and prodded daily, so, you can feel very alone. And you constantly question and blame yourself for not being able to do something so basic and natural.

I spent four years unable to explain how I felt, so it was easier to just suppress it – until my last failed IVF. I'd been in Singapore for four months for IVF. My husband was with me for the first two weeks and that was the first time he saw what I'd been going through for four years, not because he didn't want to, but because he couldn't take all that time off work.

A week or so after my transfer, I got really sick. I couldn't sit, I couldn't stand up, I was extremely lightheaded, and couldn't keep my eyes open. My husband had gone back to Doha, but luckily, I was staying with his cousins who were kind enough to tolerate me for that long. They ended up calling my husband and asking him to come as soon as possible because I wasn't looking good. I think seeing me like that was the first time he realized the toll this entire process took on me.

My result from that cycle showed that I had become pregnant, but my HCG levels were slowly dropping due to an unexplained infection which meant that the pregnancy wasn't going to hold. I was a wreck, to say the least. I tried to keep it together and to put up a strong front but this time, I just couldn't. I cried every time I thought about it, every time I talked about it; I cried even when I didn't think I was thinking about it. I had anxiety throughout the four years, but this time I got severe anxiety to the point that I felt like I couldn't breathe.

I remember the day that I couldn't ignore it anymore. I was sitting in my bathroom gasping for air and I just couldn't stop crying. I'd never felt like that before in my life and I pray that I never feel that way again. I remember praying to God asking him to take that gut-wrenching feeling away. I had been living in physical pain because of my endometriosis for years but I'd take that any day over this. I just felt so helpless with no control over myself.

A few months down the line the topic of 'the next IVF' came up and my husband who'd now seen me go through hell and back was extremely supportive throughout. He told me that I didn't have to do it again and that he was okay with not having kids if it was this stressful for me. As much as I wanted to give up, I just couldn't. I told my husband I'd try one more time.

It was time for me to go back for my next and possibly last IVF. I was on an insane diet to lose the weight that I'd gained from my previous cycle and I'd followed the diet so obsessively that I took my meals along with me to my cousins' wedding events. I needed to give this one-hundred-and-fifty per cent and I needed to know that my failed IVFs weren't because of something that I could control, which also meant that I needed to concentrate on my mental health as well.

I did everything I could possibly think of to keep myself sane. I kept reminding myself that if it didn't work and I didn't have kids, I'd still be okay because this was something I WANTED, not something I NEEDED. I swam, I walked and took in the fresh air. I made my daily trip down to Sephora and Starbucks, and I spent time with my parents who were there through all my IVF transfers.

I prayed ... A LOT! And even though I'd always prayed, I changed the way I prayed this time. Instead of hysterically saying the million duas that people sent me, I picked the one that felt closest to my heart and repeated it calmly after every prayer. Instead of asking God to give us a child or make me pregnant, I asked God to do whatever was in our best interest while praying that having a child was in our best interest. I concentrated on feeling good and being in a good headspace. I won't lie, I was still nervous and anxious, but I didn't let it take over me this time.

My doctor in Singapore was amazing. He figured that what happened to me last time could have been my body rejecting my husband's DNA, so he gave me a soybean drip before my transfer which would naturally help my body accept the embryo by fighting the antibodies, rather than giving me more meds. After my transfer, I continued to concentrate on what made ME happy. I listened only to my doctor. I ignored all other advice, such as people constantly telling me to lie down, be on bed rest, stop going out ... I did what I felt like doing. My doctor said it was counterproductive to be on bed rest and that I should go about my life normally and that's exactly what I did. I blocked everyone out, and that was the best decision I made.

On day twelve after every transfer, I'd start to bleed, and I can never forget that feeling. You feel like your heart has dropped to your knees, you're taken over by panic and confusion and you're still holding on to some sort of hope that this is just a freak incident, and it might still work. I lived in constant fear of day twelve and here it was again.

I had a few spotting episodes that same week and my doctor increased my hormone dosage in the hopes that it would help the embryo stick. On day twelve, I woke up with the fear that I was going to start bleeding and that the hormones were just delaying the inevitable. I waited the entire day and held my breath every time I went to the bathroom, but day twelve ended and I had somehow made it through. One part of me felt like this was a sign it had worked, while another part of me felt like I was just kidding myself.

It was finally day fourteen – time for my blood test – which I'd done early in the morning. I waited the entire day anxiously for the result. I still remember the moment I got the call while we were at the dinner table. The nurse said, "congratulations, your result is positive". I honestly hadn't registered what happened and when I repeated what she said, I saw my husband and his cousins jumped up, and there were lots of hugs and lots of tears. I was finally pregnant! Alhamdulillah! The hard part was finally over. I just had to get through my first trimester.

Every pregnancy is precious, but an IVF pregnancy is not only precious, it's also considered high risk. I spent my entire first trimester praying that nothing would go wrong while taking four different hormones to help my pregnancy continue.

I was so afraid that this was too good to be true that I didn't tell most of the people in my life about my pregnancy till the very end. I had a few scares when I was almost certain it wasn't going to last. There were times I had bleeding and times that I didn't feel my baby move all day. I remember I had planned a shoot and the night before I started spotting. I felt so helpless. All I could do was lay in bed crying and praying that my baby would be okay.

Other than these few incidents, my pregnancy was amazing, because I did it my way. I'd ignored everyone who told me to be on bed rest and listened only to my doctor who insisted I stay active, and honestly, that's what kept me sane.

People worry about their body during pregnancy, but I enjoyed my weight gain and my stretchmarks. I didn't feel self-conscious at all. Mothers-to-be can be frustrated with the nausea and vomiting, which I didn't have much of, but when I did have it, I didn't mind. The fact that Covid hit during my pregnancy definitely caused some anxiety, and to top it off, I was extremely upset that our families couldn't be there for my delivery and to meet our baby girl after praying for this moment for years. But as I said, I'd waited and prayed for this for years and I wasn't going to let anything ruin it for me. I was going to enjoy every minute of it, and I did. Alhamdulillah.

Maria @mariainstaglam

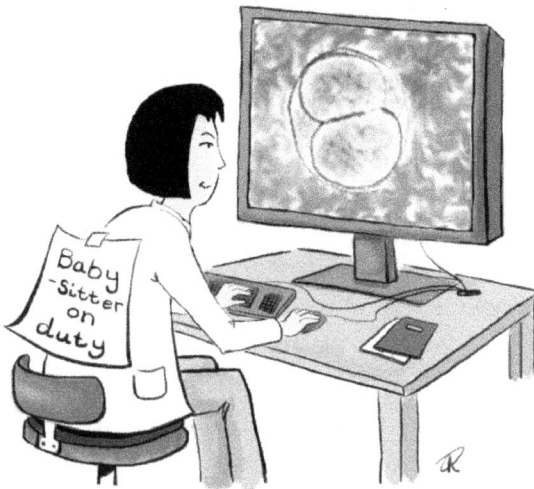

The embryologist is the first babysitter for a baby conceived via in-vitro fertilisation

Chronic illness and infertility (IVF)

I was diagnosed with endometriosis stage 4 in 2007 after years of excruciating pain during my teenage years. Endometriosis is where tissue that is similar to the lining of the womb attaches itself to organs outside of the womb, usually in the pelvis and abdomen. Stage 4 includes scar tissue and ovarian cysts. I had three diagnostic laparoscopies (keyhole surgery to look at the womb lining) over six years, and for various reasons, no endometriosis was removed.

During a menstrual period in 2012, I tried to get out of bed one morning, but couldn't; the endometriosis had caused bowel obstruction and a right pneumothorax (a collapsed lung). In hospital, emergency teams had to drain over a litre of fluid from my chest and I had a stoma for an entire year (an opening on the abdomen from the bowel). It was at this time that I was referred to an endometriosis centre for specialist treatment. The consultants informed me that IVF (in-vitro fertilisation) would be my best option to conceive. At twenty-five years old, I wasn't aware of what that entailed and wasn't ready to start a family. I also wasn't eligible for NHS (National Health Service) funded treatment at that point either.

In 2017, my husband and I began our IVF journey after trying naturally for a year. I was now eligible for three IVF cycles on the NHS. We didn't know anyone who was going through the process and it was quite lonely. After what felt like countless injections, eighteen eggs were retrieved, one blastocyst (a five-day-old fertilised egg) was transferred, and eight embryos were frozen. I wasn't expecting a positive pregnancy test as I'd been in so much pain. One line appeared on the pregnancy test and soon after I was admitted to hospital with ovarian hyperstimulation syndrome (OHSS – all the hormone medications cause the ovaries to swell). In a follow-up appointment with my endometriosis centre in London, it was confirmed through a scan that I had adenomyosis (when the inner lining of the womb breaks through its muscular wall).

Following this traumatic experience, we took a break from treatment, travelled around Europe, and got married. In the summer of 2018, we did our first frozen embryo transfer (FET). After the two-week wait, two pink lines appeared on the pregnancy test! We were absolutely delighted! We started to think about our future as parents. Even better, I was pregnant at the same time as two of my closest friends. My husband and I travelled to the clinic for our first scan, but something wasn't right. The nurse couldn't see the embryo. She ushered us into another room and suddenly, five medical professionals were staring at the monitor looking concerned. I knew something was wrong and shortly afterwards, they informed us that the pregnancy was ectopic (where the embryo develops in the fallopian tube).

We had to make our way straight to the clinic's sister hospital.

The next day I had surgery to remove the fallopian tube and pregnancy. There were complications due to the endometriosis and I was in the operating theatre for five or six hours. Fortunately, I didn't lose my ovary. But just like that, our pregnancy was over.

The grief came in waves as each year friends announced their pregnancy news. We recognised that certain situations were triggering for us and chose to withdraw from events such as baby showers. We tried to distract ourselves with work and weekends away, but it was constantly on our minds.

In 2019, we did another two frozen embryo transfers. Sadly, the embryos didn't stick. The hormones caused me to have breathing difficulties and several hospital admissions. This led to a thoracic and diaphragmatic endometriosis diagnosis. In December 2019, I underwent major surgery to repair the damage to my right lung and diaphragm. The recovery took time as I spent twelve days in hospital; my lung collapsed after surgery and I got a severe infection.

We reflected on our fertility journey in 2020 and considered that moving to a different clinic could give us a better chance. We had consultations and initial tests, but unfortunately, due to Covid-19 and my history of adenomyosis, and endometriosis, and being a BAME woman, the new clinic decided I was too high risk and couldn't offer us the treatment we wanted. With three embryos left at the NHS clinic, we opted to do a fifth transfer. Frustratingly, there was no implantation success. It was particularly difficult as we held on to hope and longed for some positive news amid the pandemic. Soon after this, two other couples close to us announced their pregnancy news.

At times it felt like a never-ending cycle. The NHS were brilliant in spotting and removing the ectopic pregnancy but just one out of five transfers resulted in a positive pregnancy test. We didn't feel anything further could be done and counselling was only offered after the last transfer. Hopes and dreams were constantly dashed, and a little piece of my heart broke every time I saw a negative result. The whole process has taken its toll on my body, leaving me with chronic illnesses and affecting my mental health.

With one frozen embryo left, we decided to move to a third fertility clinic that specialised in implantation failure. We're still holding on to hope and faith that we'll get to meet our rainbow baby. For now, we're being patient as we start the process again. Surrogacy and egg donation are also options that we're open to in the future. Looking back, I wish I'd known that the NHS funded treatment could have been used at private fertility clinics.

I'm grateful for my incredibly supportive and loving husband. He's been there every step of the way and we always make time to communicate our feelings and lift each other up. I have close relationships with family and friends. They always supported me back when I had the surgery for endometriosis. It felt natural to discuss it with them as I knew it could end up being a huge part of my life. I've never felt judgement when disclosing my journey and struggles, just love and support.

I know that whatever the outcome of IVF, I am loved. Whether

I am childfree or become a parent, there will always be more to me than that. During the pandemic, one of the most positive experiences has been becoming a part of the online community for endometriosis and infertility. I no longer feel alone in my IVF journey.

Nadine Gerin @nadinendoivf

Our dream of having a perfect family (miscarriages)

Pastor Jerry and his wife Karabo Zwane from Gauteng South Africa dreamt of having a perfect family. Little did they know they had a bumpy road ahead.

Jerry and I got married in our early twenties and neither of us ever envisioned having fertility challenges. It was actually a foreign subject to us as Jerry had a son from a previous relationship, and no-one from either of our families had fertility issues. We were on contraceptives for four years, so we could complete our studies and give ourselves time to enjoy the honeymoon stage.

Excited about starting a family, I stopped using contraceptives, hoping I'd be pregnant soon. After a year of trying, I was admitted to hospital with terrible period pains. As part of the routine tests, we had a huge surprise. "Your pregnancy test came back positive, but you've miscarried", said the doctor. I spent two days in hospital under observation, witnessing the child I so longed for bleed onto a sanitary pad. I left the hospital heartbroken, but at the same time, hopeful of the possibility of falling pregnant again soon. I wondered if I'd done something to cause the miscarriage, so I decided to look after myself.

A few months afterwards, I consulted my doctor again after experiencing another abnormally painful period. "Another miscarriage," he said. This was by far the most heart-breaking and confusing time of my life. I'd never experienced so much pain. And how did this happen when I did everything right? We prayed and even bought a few baby clothes. I was devastated.

Pressure from society and relatives started to take its toll on us. The expectation of Makoti, (Zulu Bride) not being able to bear an heir to carry the family name was a disgrace. Infertility is very much taboo in Africa, and a lot of couples still experience shame around it. My in-laws suggested that my husband should take a second wife who could bear children for him.

Further tests were conducted, and it was found that Jerry had an abnormal sperm morphology (size, shape and appearance of the sperm), and I had an auto-immune disease called Anti-phospholipid syndrome, which was the cause of the recurring early pregnancy losses. Jerry accepted his diagnosis because of his value system that emphasizes the relationship of the couple rather than being defined by children. And his faith helped him remember that all things are possible. Even though he already had a child, Jerry believed that being fertile once doesn't mean you're always fertile as anything can happen along the way. There are lifestyle and injury factors that should be considered.

I've already shared that infertility is a taboo subject in our culture, and when the cause is from the male side, it's even more taboo, so we didn't share the diagnosis with many people, except close friends. The medical professionals assured us that with the correct medication and precautionary measures such as avoiding very hot showers – both of which Jerry was extremely diligent about – the situation could be turned around.

We were both put on medication to increase our chances and also to keep the pregnancy. We tried artificial insemination (AI – where sperm is introduced into the cervix) twice without success. Depression got the better of us and we stopped trying. We were no longer mindful of ovulation and figuring out pregnancy symptoms. We finally accepted that we may never have children but were still devoted to having a happy marriage.

After years of struggling with infertility, we conceived naturally, and I was immediately given medication which I injected daily for the duration of my pregnancy. On the 1st January 2012, I gave birth to a healthy baby boy and we experienced the joy of an answered prayer. But just when we thought infertility was a thing of the past, after our son was born, we had three further miscarriages, and an ectopic pregnancy (where the pregnancy develops in the fallopian tube and is life-threatening).

We've used our journey to help couples who need support, and also to raise awareness about infertility through our organisation called 'Hannah – You Are Not Alone'.

Karabo Zwane @hannah_youarenotalone

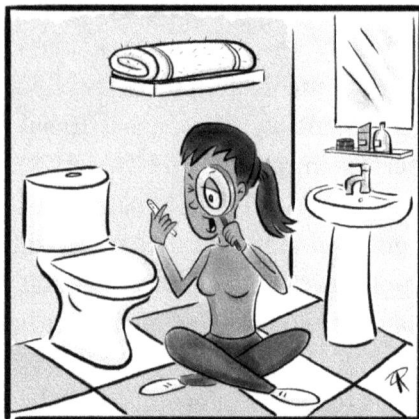

"I can definitely see a 2nd pink line"

Carry on, let go and don't talk about it (baby loss)

One in two people in the UK will be diagnosed with cancer in their lifetime.

One in seven couples will be affected by infertility in the UK.

One in four pregnancies ends in loss in the UK. And these figures are similar around the world.

These statistics matter because I'm affected by all three. I was diagnosed with womb cancer in March 2017, along with a diagnosis of blocked fallopian tubes, rendering me infertile. I can't have children without medical intervention – IVF (In-Vitro Fertilisation) in my case. My first successful IVF cycle ended in the loss of my daughter, Jaya, at twenty-two weeks and one-day gestation. My second cycle ended in a failed transfer, so that was a loss of my perfectly graded embryo or embaby as they are sometimes referred to in the IVF community.

I thought I'd dealt pretty well with my cancer and infertility diagnosis. My family is quite open-minded and were proud of me when I shared my cancer story with a Gynaecological cancer charity and a newspaper. They asked a lot about the next steps, IVF etc and they were ecstatic when I announced my pregnancy.

Fast forward to losing Jaya and I've mostly been met with silence. The Indian community isn't on the whole very good at dealing with or talking about death or anything hard. Their attitude is carry on, let go, and don't talk about it. It's too uncomfortable and they don't want to feel that way. I found this difficult to fathom when people had been so supportive of my previous struggles.

When Jaya died there was an influx of support; visits to the hospital where she was born, attendance at my parent's house on the day of her funeral and the following weeks after. Then it stopped. Then she was forgotten about, as was I. The family who I thought would always be there – my extended family and some of my husband's immediate family – were nowhere to be seen. Any mention of Jaya was met with silence, but new babies being born, birthdays and other occasions were celebrated while Jaya was completely ignored.

In the first few weeks, I can honestly say I tried to ignore what had happened and be strong and carry on. And the people who were in contact were a welcome distraction. However, after the initial shock had worn off when real-life resumed, I desperately needed the support of my nearest and dearest. Sadly, they preferred that I forget about my baby and made that clear by ignoring my Facebook posts, WhatsApp messages and Instagram comments whenever I mentioned her name. It was hurtful and unfair. Silence is by far the worst reaction to the loss of a baby, but other things have been difficult too. I've been told:

"Let go."

"It's not healthy to still be like this."

"You'll feel better when you have another one."

"At least you know you can get pregnant."

The only conclusion I can come to is that people don't think before they speak. But if they truly thought for a second, how would they feel if these things were said to them. I'm sure they wouldn't appreciate them either. That's the issue.

Another thing that took me by surprise the day after Jaya died was when my husband drove back to Preston to get some of our things. I only had maternity clothes with me and didn't feel like I could wear them anymore. He called me to say that his aunt had told them that his pregnant sister-in-law shouldn't visit me. I was shocked and hurt. I'd already been punished by losing my daughter, and now I was being punished for bad luck as if baby loss was contagious. This is the biggest issue with the Indian culture – it makes you feel that if you've lost a baby, you are now tainted. You can't take part in pregnancy ceremonies or birth celebrations for someone else because you're deemed unlucky. I don't know who made up these rules, but they're ridiculous.

I've been extremely vocal about my experience of losing Jaya because I feel the Indian community needs to change with the times, not stay stuck in the dark ages. I wouldn't want anyone to feel the isolation and hurt that I've felt in the last fourteen months, and continue to feel. The statistics speak for themselves – one in four pregnancies. That means someone you know will have experienced the horror of pregnancy loss. They shouldn't have to feel shame and loneliness on top of that, because the Indian community thinks they should remain silent. So, if you're feeling alone and you have no support, please reach out. I will always listen. You are not alone.

All my love,

Vaish x

Vaishali Bamania @jayas_star

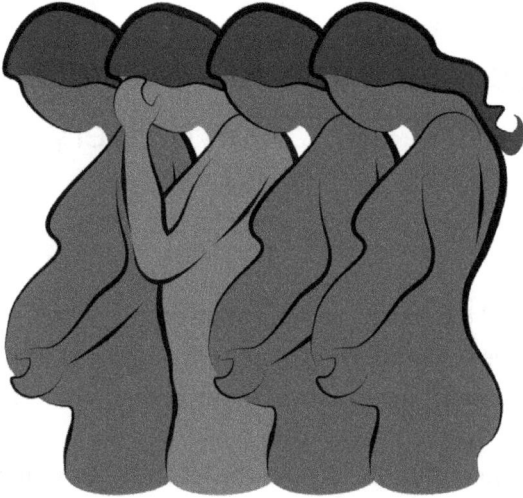

1 in 4 pregnancies sadly result in miscarriage/pregnancy loss

My secondary infertility was due to my first Caesarean delivery

I always find it funny when someone asks me to "tell my story". It didn't seem like much of a story at all when I was living it, and sometimes it feels more of a dream than my reality.

It began when my college sweetheart and I got married right after college. We'd discussed having children before and even picked out their names, but life had other plans. After being married for about six months, my husband wanted to start our family. At first, I was on board, but deep down I felt that I wasn't ready to become a mom. I'd always had a gnawing feeling that I may have issues conceiving, due to my cycles being painful, heavy and feeling constantly nauseous. Nothing seemed to help, despite multiple doctor visits where I was given birth control without any tests being done. So, I was scared to try out of fear that something might happen.

We started to try, but then I decided that things were moving way too fast and I told my husband that I no longer wanted to try for a baby now. I took a break from it all and instead focused on taking charge of my health and body.

In January of 2009, we went on a Daniel Fast – a Bible fast with our church, where you eat a plant-based diet, plus I began drinking red raspberry leaf tea daily. I drank more water, exercised four times a week with my husband and ate more fruit and vegetables rather than processed foods. I noticed that I was sleeping better and my skin was glowing. I wasn't eating meat, so I guess my body began to heal itself because I'd had one of the best menstrual cycles I'd ever had – less blood loss, no clots, and a lot less pain. I continued drinking red raspberry leaf tea with a hint of honey daily, and in February I conceived!

It was a total shock to me because I thought that I couldn't get pregnant, due to my heavy, painful periods. Yet here I was staring at two lines on a pregnancy test. My husband was elated, but I went from shock to dread because my anxiety got the better of me. I'd got pregnant so easily even though I had all these problems with my periods ... so, of course, something had to be wrong with my baby, right?

Waiting for my first ultrasound felt like it took a thousand years; my husband sensed that I was pregnant the night our daughter was conceived, so, waiting for another month before I could see the doctor while worrying that something was off, seemed like torture. As my husband and I entered the room to hear our baby's heartbeat I held my breath just in case they didn't find one. The ultrasound technician showed us the most amazingly beautiful little blob on that screen, and from that day on I fell in love with my little peanut (that's what we called her until we found out that she was a girl), and I worried daily for her safety.

My pregnancy was uneventful and lasted nine months and two

139

days. I was never sick, and I didn't have swollen feet or an achy back. However, I did gain about fifty pounds, but most of it was in my belly. As an avid researcher, I watched all the documentaries that I could, read books and scanned articles. I then decided on having a midwife because I wanted a natural and medication-free birth.

On November 3rd, 2009, I entered the hospital to be induced because my baby had, 'run out of room and was too big to remain inside'. When I got there the nurse informed me that I was already in labor but I was given some medication to help me sleep, along with Cervadil, a medication to relax and open the cervix, even though I was already three centimeters dilated. This wasn't anything like I'd planned, but I didn't know anything about giving birth so I trusted the midwife.

After eleven hours of natural labor and thirty minutes of pushing, I was told that my baby's heart rate was dropping, so I needed a Caesarean delivery. I was wheeled into OR where my daughter was born and my life from then on would never be the same. During the delivery, the doctor found severe scarring all over my uterus, fallopian tubes, bowel, and ovaries. She decided to help by scraping away the scarred tissue so that I'd be able to conceive in future, and then told me I was lucky to have been able to conceive at all.

Healing from the C-section proved to be extremely challenging. My body went into shock and each time I ate, the food would come back out one end or the other. At about six months postpartum, I developed a cyst in my right breast and a cyst on my right ovary. I researched once again and began healing my body through nutrition and supplements and was able to get rid of the cysts. I thought that my body was functioning properly until our daughter was about three years old and we tried again. Up till this point, we hadn't been trying to prevent pregnancy, but nothing had happened. Since things were easy the first time, we thought there wouldn't be any issues this time either, but we were WRONG.

My cycles began coming every two weeks. I started having hot flashes, and I generally felt off and tired all the time. After a year of nothing happening, we went to see a fertility specialist who told me that my eggs were old, my tubes were blocked, and there was nothing he could do other than IVF (in-vitro fertilisation). I was twenty-seven years old. My AMH level, (a blood test used by some doctors to estimate the number of follicles, and therefore eggs, inside the ovaries) was 0.7 which is considered low, and my thyroid numbers were also low. I was also in excruciating pain each month during ovulation since having given birth, but no one wanted to listen. We had no money, our credit wasn't great, and we needed twenty thousand dollars to have a baby. I was completely devastated and sank into a deep depression.

I told my husband that I understood if he left me because we wanted three kids and I couldn't have any more. He replied: "I love you and we have a child, but even if we didn't, you are enough." Somehow his words meant nothing because all I heard was that I was a failure, and my body was broken. As I wallowed in self-pity, a lightbulb in my head came on, and I decided that I'd prove the doctor wrong. That's when my obsession with healing my body began. For the next five years, I worked hard at eating well, tried natural therapies, took supplements, did acupuncture, and had fertility massages.

In 2015, we decided to adopt, so that we could have children that were closer to our daughter's age, while we prepared for IVF. That process was long and hard with its own battles, but in the end, we became parents to two more children. They were never meant to replace the babies that I couldn't have, and somehow, I knew they never could, so, I compartmentalized that experience and put it into a separate box, while continuing to plan for another baby.

In 2016, I sought the help of the doctor who'd performed my C-section because she seemed to be the only person that was willing to listen to me. She sent me to see a specialist who was certain he could help me. They did a Hysterosalpingogram, (HSG, an x-ray to check if the fallopian tubes are open and if the inside of the womb is normal), which showed no signs of scarring but only one of my tubes appeared to be open. I decided to have surgery to open the tube, but when I woke up, I was told that both my fallopian tubes had to be removed as they'd been damaged during my C-section. All the years I spent blaming myself and feeling broken was because of my C-section, where the scar tissue was removed without my consent. I was both hurt and relieved because I finally had an answer as to why I spent all those years in excruciating pain – but now, my only opportunity to conceive was through IVF and we still didn't have the money.

Since I had to wait to do IVF, I decided to do something else to occupy my time. So later that year, I became a birth doula and began supporting families. It was a dream come true because it allowed me to advocate for others and find healing in knowing that I was making a difference.

In 2018, we finally had enough money to seek help so I went to a fertility doctor to end the journey that started so long ago. Then a series of unfortunate events happened. First, my doctor passed away which meant I had to see a different doctor and wait for an appointment. Then my test results were never released to me. Lastly, the clinic office staff never returned my calls and I decided that enough was enough. My husband had already decided that he didn't want to have more children, but I was still hoping to have more.

However, when I reflected on the horrible experience with my clinic, I began to support others as a fertility coach, and that's how Ultimatefertilityconsultant was born. And in 2019, I started my non-profit organization, 'Faithfully Fertile Foundation' that provides education, emotional and financial support to those dealing with infertility. My story didn't end with a baby, but it did help me to give birth to my purpose and help others on their journey to parenthood.

Dr Sierra Bizzell @ultimatefertilityconsultant

My heterotopic pregnancy experience (pregnancy loss)

I had a chemical pregnancy (miscarriage before the fifth week of pregnancy) early in my marriage. Dr Google was my consultant at the time and I quickly diagnosed myself and understood what happened. Months into my life as a newlywed, I'd made calls to a fertility clinic asking if I should be worried and specifically referenced my previous loss. But I was advised early losses are common and I should try again after a few months, then if there was no pregnancy, I could come in for a consultation.

I got pregnant a few weeks after the call to the clinic with a BFP (big fat positive; positive result on a home pregnancy test). I remember being elated, jumping and dancing around. And then, suddenly, I stopped – oh my, was I jumping too high? Or was the dancing too much for the baby? Random thoughts raced through my mind. If you stay around me long enough, you'll soon realise I have a serious case of OCD, but that's a conversation for another day.

My Darling Husband (DH) was due to come home, so I quickly made a makeshift card with the words: 'Guess Who's Going to Be A Daddy?' He was thrilled when he saw it and we were quick to thank the Heavens for this blessing. We were soon discussing baby names and which hospital would be best to have the baby.

A few weeks after that, I experienced some bleeding and had to go to the clinic where an ultrasound was done and I was admitted for a couple of days for monitoring. Afterwards, I was asked to go home and remain on bed rest. Everything seemed fine at that point.

Not long afterwards, my DH had to travel, so, I proceeded to stay with my mum as I didn't want to be alone. It was fun spending time there and getting pampered; just bed rest, lots of food and watching movies. I could see the weight gain coming on quickly, but it was okay, gaining weight while pregnant isn't frowned upon. It's expected anyways.

But as my weight increased so did the unease in my spirit. I felt something was weird and I remember discussing it with my mum and saying, I think I should go to the clinic. Of course, my mum being the religious person she is, proceeded to call a Pastor who then prayed and warned of unnecessary clinic visits. After all, there weren't any obvious issues; it all seemed to be in my head.

But I still felt a sense of unrest and discussed my thoughts with one of my sisters who advised me to go to the clinic. But after weighing up the conversations, I figured I should probably wait a few more days and see how I felt.

I awoke one morning around 3 a.m. I hadn't been asleep for long as I'd spent the previous night playing a praise and worship song I'd just discovered. As I mentioned earlier, I do have OCD and I must have played the same song on repeat for around two hours! I felt uneasy and the more I asked God to take it away, the worse it became. I instinctively knew I should go to the clinic.

I got dressed, and my mum woke up and asked what I was doing. I told her I was going to the clinic, and of course, she told me to back to bed and not panic. But I called her driver and asked him to come over. This was now around 4 a.m. My mum wasn't impressed with my impulsiveness but agreed to come along.

On arrival at the clinic, I was taken to the examination room and asked why I came in. I told them, I just felt uneasy. Some blood tests were taken, and I was kept on the bed till the gynaecologist showed up a few hours later. He asked me what the issue was and my reason for coming to the clinic. By this time, I was felt much better, so I asked if I could return home. Luckily, he declined and stated that he'd rather get some blood work and more scans done.

Looking back now, I realise he must have been God-sent. My haemoglobin was dropping each time the blood test was done and I collapsed after getting up from the scan. When I awoke, I was surrounded by doctors and nurses all obviously panicked. The scan had shown fluid around my abdomen and chest region. All these factors taken together were pointing to a potential issue, but I wasn't in pain, which wasn't usual and didn't align with the other symptoms.

I was moved back to the examination room and the doctor came to speak with me saying he wanted to perform surgery to check what was going on internally. All this time, my mum was still in the waiting room and asking after me, wondering what was going on. I asked them to inform her that I was doing well, but needed to get some rest, warning them not to tell her I was having surgery. I certainly didn't need the drama at that time. After much discussion with my DH, we decided to proceed with the surgery and committed it all into God's hands.

The lights went out and when I regained consciousness, I discovered I'd had a heterotopic pregnancy – a twin pregnancy with one embryo in the fallopian tube and another in the uterus. I'd been bleeding internally for so long that I needed multiple blood transfusions. I'd lost a tube and both my babies. The uterine pregnancy was masking the other pregnancy in the tube; doctors were able to see the pregnancy in the uterus so didn't check anywhere else. As a result of my experience, I now advocate for early scans and for them to include checks on the tubes and the uterus, even if there is a uterine pregnancy.

Despite my devastating loss, I was thankful that I was alive and well, thankful that God had saved me and given me another chance at life. The loss was overwhelming, and I experienced PTSD (post-traumatic stress disorder) afterwards. But every day I awoke and witnessed another sunrise, I was grateful for another day. Like Sean Stephenson, the motivational speaker and author says: "If you have a heartbeat, there's still time for your dreams," and I'm still holding on to that …

Ola @thefertilityconversations and @fertilityconversations

There's no healing in silence (miscarriage and stillbirth)

"How long have you been married?" If you've ever been asked that question, you know what's coming next, don't you? "No kids yet?" "What are you waiting for?" "You should have your kids while you're still young!" "You can't keep putting your career first!"

I heard these comments for four years at every wedding and family function I went to. I'd smile a reluctant smile at the random Aunty who felt it her place to probe, judge and amplify my childless status. I'd wish for someone to come and rescue me, pray for the ground to swallow me up. But most of the time I stood there and endured the lecture. I had something to say in response, but the words just never came out. What I wanted to say was: "Aunty, you don't know what I'm going through, please stop. Your words are killing me. PLEASE stop!" What Aunty didn't know was that we were trying for a family. We longed for a child. In fact, we'd been pregnant, many, many times. But every time we miscarried; I was silently dealing with heartbreak after heartbreak after heartbreak.

Six miscarriages and one stillbirth later, I decided enough was enough. This is when my blog, 'A Drug Named Hope' was born. I decided to break all the unwritten rules in our community – to speak up; to share my story; to challenge the voices around us, and to do it publicly. Breaking my own silence did something to me. It freed me. I released the weight I was carrying. And can you guess what happened next? I got pregnant for the eighth time. And against all odds, this pregnancy went the distance. I gave birth to my first living baby.

Did breaking my silence have a role to play in my only successful pregnancy? I have no scientific proof, but in my heart of hearts, I believe it did play a significant role. It helped me heal from the inside out. Speaking out about my miscarriages helped me release all my bottled-up emotions and helped me come to terms with all that I'd been through. Putting pen to paper allowed me to explore my feelings more deeply, process them and heal from within. And by making my story public, I also silenced the Auntie's too!

There's no healing in silence. We aren't taught how to process our pain and heal from our trauma. Instead, as a community, we're encouraged to keep quiet, to bottle it up and to put on a brave face. But beneath the façade is often raw, raging, emotion. Like a pressure cooker, the more we keep that emotion suppressed, the more the pressure builds. By keeping a lid on it, it won't just disappear, it won't miraculously dissipate. And left unattended, the pressure will continue to build until it's too much to contain. It will erupt. Uncontrollably. And without warning. The strong emotions need to go somewhere. They need to be released. We need to hit the release value. So, my advice to anyone experiencing the pain, the grief, the trauma of miscarriage, of stillbirth, of baby loss...

Release the pressure valve

- Honour your feelings – Permit yourself to feel whatever it is you need to feel. Go into the discomfort of the emotion. Don't push it away, like we're taught to. Allow it in. There's no shame in feeling difficult emotions. Feel them and let them pass through you.

- Process your thoughts – Get yourself a journal or spill out your emotions on your laptop and start writing about everything you're thinking and feeling. Don't judge or dismiss anything. Don't worry about grammar or technicalities. Just write. And keep writing. This is for your eyes only; you don't need to share your writing with anyone. See it as an opportunity to acknowledge and put down the thoughts that run wild in your mind.

- Talk to someone – reach out to someone you trust, see your GP, request counselling, join a support group. Break your silence, talk about your experience, and feel the deep release that comes with it. Allow yourself to be supported by people who 'get it' and are there to help you heal. You don't need to go through this alone.

- Find your voice – as you go through the stages above – beware, you may well find a roaring voice within that wants to confront the Aunty who dares to pry into your business!

Remember you're not alone and you will get through this. You may not recognise the person you become, but my goodness you'll be so deeply proud of her. I know I am.

Gurinder Mann @adrugnamedhope

My journey to motherhood through surrogacy

Shared on the Nairaland Forum in May 2020

Thirteen years ago, aged twenty-two, I married right after university, without the wisdom to realise the importance of finding my feet first. My husband was eleven years older than me. He wasn't rich but I thought we loved each other. During my Youth Service Year, I conceived, but sadly, I lost the baby soon after.

Hubby was helped to get a stable government job by my family. When I lost my first pregnancy, we were staying with his parents for a few months, due to our financial situation. While my husband was traveling for work, my father-in-law said, "Did your ladies in the water say to you that the day you give birth, you would die?"

With the new job we were soon able to move back home and continued our lives. Three more miscarriages came along with many dramas, ranging from deliverances to traditional midwives to my in-law's commanding our home.

Finally, one day almost five years later, my husband was again away from home, and his father called my aunty to tell her, "They don't want to marry their daughter again". I was at work when aunty broke the news to me. I travelled that night to the in-laws with my aunty and grandmother to beg that we remain married. We were not given an audience. They didn't even open their gate, despite being able to see my husband's car in the compound.

At 9 p.m. my companions begged me to go home with them. I refused and chose to spend the night in a shed close by. The was no electricity in the neighbourhood, everywhere was dark. At midnight, the power was restored, and in the shed where I was hiding, I saw my father-in-law walking round the compound spraying incense, (he attended celestial church). I called out to him, "Daddy, Daddy!" I knew he heard me but he behaved as if I was a ghost.

At that point, I knew I was wasting my time. I started trekking. I trekked to the motor park which was a long distance away. Vigilantes stopped me numerous times on the way, but my tearful face ensured they left me alone. I travelled back home and resumed work while praying and fasting for my husband's return. Mehn! I lost weight without even trying.

One day, I realized I might have the password to hubby's Facebook. I tried it and it worked. What I saw caused me pain, but it also gave me strength knowing the breakup wasn't because of anything he was accusing me of — such as saying a pastor revealed I was sent into his life by the kingdom of darkness to destroy him. To this, I asked him if the kingdom of darkness also gave out jobs? He said he repaid me, because the kingdom of darkness connected me back to the job I'd been doing before, even though it didn't last. Oh, and he wanted me to pay my salary to him by the way.

At this point, I got some courage to begin living again and applied for a divorce. To this, he also said, "Good wives wait for their husbands, no matter how long they're gone for." But not me, I wanted to go ahead with the divorce, because I wanted to eventually remarry.

When we got to the court, my husband was accompanied by his father. They claimed that hubby didn't abscond, but that I did! I guess they were afraid I'd want compensation. Walking out of court, his father waved at me and I wondered why. He was barely divorced when he remarried, and now has kids. Things went sour with my place of work and I relocated to a bigger city and that was my fresh start.

I met my current husband two years after the divorce. I hid nothing from him, especially my challenges with infertility. We married that same year and I got pregnant and miscarried. In our second pregnancy, I was given a *cerclage*, (a stitch in the cervix to close it during pregnancy), yet the pregnancy still ended. I almost ended along with it as my body went into shock due to its inability to dispel the dead foetus, because of the cerclage.

After eight pregnancy losses at fourteen weeks, I visited more hospitals, met insensitive, money-mad doctors, but finally, a correct diagnosis was made after having a hysteroscopy (a medical procedure that looks inside the womb). My womb was just too small to carry to term; it wasn't expanding with the pregnancies. But I had no demons worrying me. Getting a diagnosis, at last, was some sort of relief. "What can we do doctor?" I asked. The doctor said, "Have you considered adoption?" I was shattered. I went home and discussed it with my husband. We agreed to adopt and started the application.

Soon after, I was on social media and saw someone advertising that they needed a surrogate, and like a lightbulb, the idea stuck. I wrote to the woman and we started chatting. One day she posted that she needed someone to donate blood for a relative of hers. Although she was still an online stranger who I'd never met, I offered.

That was the first day I met my good friend Mrs R. I then put up an advert for a surrogate as I couldn't afford the prices the agencies were charging. After two bad experiences, I finally found a good person that we could afford. And God somehow ensured the money came.

When God wants to turn your story around, you know it's your time. I paid for one IVF (in-vitro fertilization) cycle at the hospital we'd been to before, but I was already looking for the money in case the first cycle didn't work. But guess what? IT WORKED! My twin daughters are now three months old.

And then we heard about our adoption application from two years ago.

I tell my story for any woman who's waiting for a similar miracle and thinks that God doesn't answer her prayers after twenty years.

@mysurrogatetwins

Ten things ... (miscarriage)

... You should NEVER hear someone say after a miscarriage

"It wasn't a proper baby."
    "You'll be fine."
    "You'll get over it."
    "It's nature's way."
    "It wasn't your time."
    "Something must have been wrong and it's probably for the best."
    "At least you can get pregnant so you can have another baby."
    "Don't worry, you can try again."
    "Everything happens for a reason."
    "Was it your fault?"

... You SHOULD hear someone say after a miscarriage

"It wasn't your fault."
    "I'm sorry for your loss."
    "If you would like to talk about it, I'm here."
    "Be gentle with yourself."
    "This is sh*t and it will be sh*t for a while, but I promise you it will get better."

"It's OK to be sad and cry."
"I know it was early but it was still your baby."
"Your baby was loved."
"It's OK to be angry for as long as you want."
"Your baby will always be with you in your heart."

Sheila Lamb @fertilitybooks

My emotional experience after the death of Damani

When Damani died, I immediately went into a black hole. The minute the doctor said his heart stopped beating in the NICU, (neonatal intensive care) I lost it. I felt like I was in a dream and needed someone to wake me up. We were asked if we wanted to hold him, which we did and we wailed. I've never seen my husband so heartbroken. That made me feel even worse. Sadly, they didn't ask us if we wanted any photos and it has been our biggest regret, because we only have one photo of him which was taken hours after he was born. They talk about mom guilt when parenting a living child, but I wish more was spoken about the guilt we parents feel after our child dies. That guilt can eat you alive and send you into depression for a very long time. It took two years, yet there are still times when I get drawn into the 'what ifs.'

After being discharged from the hospital, I was told to keep banding my breasts so that the milk wouldn't come in. To my surprise when tidying up one evening, my milk was dripping down on to my leg. I was so shocked that I let out a wail I'll never forget. It was at this moment I completely despised my body. It didn't work to keep my child alive, yet, here it was operating as if Damani was still here. My C-section scar was a painful reminder of what was and what could've been, and I still haven't fully accepted my scar as part of me.

I blamed myself and there were times I thought my husband blamed me too. I used to wonder if our marriage would survive this; would I ever be able to give him more children? Will our love ever be the same?

So many questions swirled through my mind, the emotional toll from the trauma associated with Damani's death was just too much. I remember begging God to take the pain away because I wasn't strong enough and I couldn't do it. My faith struggled, but it was in that darkness I developed a more personal relationship with God. He kept being my strength when I had nothing left.

During the midst of my pain, a month after Damani's death, I created a social media page to share his story. I was surprised by the feedback and how many others in Jamaica were struggling. I felt so alone and then I found the baby loss community, and I suddenly felt like I belonged.

I find the silence around pregnancy and infant loss unbearable. People don't see us as parents because there's no living child. And that hurts, because, although Damani isn't physically in our arms, we still parent him in our own way. We still think about him and wonder what he'd be doing now. We still feel parent guilt, wondering if we're honouring or remembering him enough by how we live our lives. The only difference is we don't get to create new memories with our child, which is why memories and validation of their existence are so important to us bereaved parents.

Sometimes it still feels like a bad dream; there were times I dreamed he was alive, but I know he's not physically here anymore, and I've accepted that. In honouring him, I've embraced life after his death, memorializing him in any way I can, as any parent should. I've been learning to be patient and kind to myself. I've realized that time doesn't necessarily heal this trauma, but time has taught me how to cope better with his death. There have been, and will be, times when it's too much to bear and all I can do is sit with my grief ... and I've been learning that's okay too.

Grief is an act of love. And I'll always love Damani, so this grief, this grief is forever. All I can do is learn to live with it.

Crystal-Gayle @4damani

Finding hope after pregnancy loss

I'm just like many other thirty-something women; I work full time as an essential worker, I'm a full-time wife and the mom of one fur-baby, our Boston Terrier, Rocky. As fulfilling as work and my home life are, my husband and I always knew long before we were married that we wanted to be parents someday. The only snare in the fantasy was the unforeseen difficulties we'd face trying to conceive.

I stopped taking birth control in March of 2017, following a vacation to Trinidad and Tobago for the Carnival. I wanted to allow adequate time to detox from the contraceptive hormones my reproductive system had been bombarded with for a decade. We figured we'd be announcing our pregnancy sometime in the next few months. Despite our best efforts to track ovulation, body temperature, cervical mucus, and use technology to bring a baby into the world, we were still a family of three, including our dog. We even had a baseline test to see if we should pursue fertility treatments.

Shortly after receiving our test results from the fertility center, we discovered that I was PREGNANT! The immediate shock and joy we felt was the single happiest day ever; June 10, 2018. It was spectacular; the sun shining brightly, the birds chirping even more beautifully, and nothing could ruin my high. Nothing that is until nearly a month later on July 4, 2018.

I began the holiday with spotting, cramping, and back pain but chalked it up to hormones and my body generally being sore because of the changes taking place. Little did I know, our ray of hope would soon be extinguished. As the day continued, the cramping continued and I was also doubled over with the worst pain I'd ever endured, losing more blood than any menstrual cycle I could remember. My husband rushed me to the hospital where my OB/GYN was on staff, after quickly leaving a family barbecue. I immediately felt panic, horror, and then the numbing realization that I was having a miscarriage. Even as the emergency room doctors and ultrasound technicians were buzzing around us, it took every ounce of self-control I could muster not to give in to the agony I felt. I finally couldn't hold my tears back any longer when my husband, Dominic, began crying in the emergency room. That broke me.

We've spent the past two years recovering from the most difficult summer of our adult lives. We found support in our group of young marrieds at church and in the friends we made in college and professional school. Very few people talk openly about miscarriage and pregnancy loss; it's stigmatized and crushing to live through. But we've found catharsis comes from transparent dialogue and embracing the roller coaster of emotions we feel daily. Most importantly, healing has come from our faith that God will give us the children we both desire someday.

Amid the COVID-19 pandemic, we've pushed our efforts to conceive even further. After a fruitless IUI (intra-uterine insemination) cycle in 2019, we elected to move forward with IVF (in-vitro fertilization) in 2020. In February we were surprised to find out that I'd an endometrioma on my right ovary (which is a common form of endometriosis where endometrial tissue is found inside and sometimes on the ovary). Worried that our goals to begin IVF would be delayed, I had an MRI scan just as the world went into lockdown due to Coronavirus. As the first wave of the pandemic wreaked havoc in the United States, my laparoscopy to remove the endometrioma was pushed to July. It was absolutely worth the wait. Reclaiming my health and living without constant endometriosis pain has been incredibly liberating. Now, as the year is quickly charging toward its close, we're preparing for our first frozen embryo transfer. We successfully underwent egg retrieval and genetic testing in October! We're praying that our transfer also goes well, and our miracle baby will join us in the Summer or Fall of 2021!

Shannon Chapman @bellewithabump

It's important to find your community (infertility & IVF)

A few years ago, I had no idea what infertility even was. I didn't know about it because it wasn't discussed. I never knew if my mother, aunts, or grandmothers dealt with issues concerning their fertility, because from my perspective as they'd had children, there wasn't a problem. At the time my husband and I were ready to grow our family, many had already started theirs ahead of us. We honestly didn't think we'd run into any obstacles since my husband already had a child almost ten years before.

Once I received my diagnosis of tubal infertility, the first thing I did was cry, but then once the tears dried up, I began to open up about the journey. As a person of faith, sharing my story was liberating. It allowed me to be honest but also to help someone else who may have gone through the same issues. One thing I came to realize was that many women weren't as open to sharing and therefore suffered in silence. Even when I went through my process, out of my beautiful journey of IVF, I connected with an amazing community of women who I could pray for, vent to, and share experiences. Eventually, it became a passion to be the voice for those who suffered silently. One of the most important things I've discovered in this tough battle of infertility is community. As I began to be more vocal, the less alone I felt. I know speaking out isn't easy, so it's crucial you open up to people you can trust, people who won't judge you, people who'll just sit and listen and be kind. This community is not one you ask to be a part of, but if you connect and network with those who share your journey, it makes it easier when you have someone to lean on.

This path has changed my life and I, for one, am very blessed because of it.

Asia B Cash @thefruitfulplace

Not talking didn't help me to cope (infertility & IVF)

Here I was staring once again at a negative pregnancy test. I've been here so many times feeling hopeless. Will this happen for us. Will it?

As a young girl, I remember reading fairy tales and all I knew was – you grow up, you meet a man, you get married, you buy a house, you have children … Not everyone marries a man, not everyone wants to get married, not everyone can buy a house and not everyone can have children. But who tells you the fairy tale is sometimes just that, a tale? Who do you talk to about this?

In the Nigerian community, infertility is a taboo subject, and no-one talks openly about it. Not talking about what you're going through doesn't help you, in fact, it's the worst thing you can do. After all I've been through over eight years – endometrial hyperplasia stage 4, (an unusually thick womb lining due to too many cells), delays to have this treated, IVF (in-vitro fertilisation), negative pregnancy tests, sperm DNA fragmentation, (abnormal genetic material in the sperm), visits to clinics in Greece, Poland and the Czech Republic looking for answers, along with elevated NK cells, (some believe these cells can cause implantation failure and pregnancy loss), I have grown and learnt so much. And remaining silent didn't help me to cope. That's why I share what I've experienced ... to help and support others.

Chi-Chi @makingbabyo_

We were told we weren't praying hard enough (IVF)

I met Yemi (one of the authors) at her Fertility forum in 2015. The speakers spoke about the different fertility treatments, relevant investigations and sperm tests. I went with my partner who's now my husband. We'd been trying for a baby for three years and were both thirty-four years old. We followed this with attending a fertility clinic and did some tests to find out if we had any fertility problems.

We also approached our pastor to inform him of our intentions, but were shocked at his reaction to our lack of faith, preferring to seek fertility treatment rather than praying more We weren't sure what to do and felt very confused as we weren't expecting to hear that.

We confided in a couple who'd been at our church as they'd had their children with the help of IVF (In-Vitro Fertilisation). They left the church because they didn't feel supported and felt they couldn't confide in anyone about their situation.

Both my Fallopian tubes were blocked so I needed IVF to conceive. Thankfully, we now have two beautiful girls and thank

God for their laughter every day. The only regret we have is that we didn't freeze our left-over embryos because we felt guilty putting our children in the freezer.

Bimbola

My partner showed no commitment (double donor conception)

My name is JO for the sake of anonymity. I was in a relationship for about five years trying to conceive, but I had to pay for the treatment as he had two children from a previous relationship. To him, I was the one with the issue. I was thirty-three at the time and informed by my private doctor that I still had some eggs, but I needed to start straight away.

So, we started the process, but my partner showed no commitment. When I told him about the appointments, he looked at me with that frown as if to say, he doesn't need to know. The injecting was very hard on me with little support from him. When I screamed sometimes, being fearful of injecting, he'd shout out: "Is this not just an injection, what is all this yelling and shouting, JO?'' I couldn't speak to anyone as no one knew I was going through infertility which made it very difficult. I was low and lonely, but thankfully Yemi (the co-author of this book), was there to listen when I was in tears.

The treatment continued till the day of egg collection. My partner said he'd meet me at the clinic as he needed to pop into work. I thought nothing of it until after I had the procedure and the embryologist kept on asking when my partner was coming in to give his sample. I called his phone but it went to voicemail. I must have left twenty messages and was crying at one point thinking, *what's going on and why has he turned off his phone?* I had to tell the embryologist that my partner was running late and then continued to cry that I didn't know what was going on. The embryologist calmed me down and went to call one of the nurses. They asked if we'd quarrelled to which I said 'nope'. I lied, but I was so stressed and just wanted him to show up. I got dressed and sat in the waiting room, hoping he'd arrive and apologise.

Long story short. He never showed up. When I saw him, his excuse was, he couldn't leave work to come to the clinic. I was numb and didn't know what to say. The relationship wasn't the same. We hardly talked afterwards.

One day, I came back from work to discover he'd moved out. He'd left a note that it wasn't working between us. I cried but was relieved in a way that I could get on with my life, although I was depressed for a while not knowing where to turn.

Fast forward, I opted to do fertility treatment on my own with donated eggs and sperm and now have a beautiful baby. I am eternally grateful to God.

JO

If you're needing to use fertility treatment to start or add to your family, we're sorry you're having to turn to science. If this will be your first cycle, understandably you're worried and apprehensive as you don't know what to expect. In Sheila's book *This is IVF and other fertility treatments: Real-life experiences of going through fertility treatments,* you'll read over thirty true stories from women and men who have themselves been through IVF and IUI treatments, some successful and some not. All our stories are different but how we feel is very similar, and their words will be sure to bring you comfort and ensure you don't feel alone. It's available as an eBook and paperback here: https://books2read.com/u/31YVp6

If you will be using IVF or IUI to start or add to your family, you will go through what is known in the infertility community as 'the dreaded two-week wait'. This is the time period between when an embryo (IVF), or sperm (IUI), has been placed in your womb and you can do a pregnancy test that is reliable. These two weeks are a rollercoaster of emotions where positivity and negativity are constant companions. Read other women's stories of how they got through this emotional time in Sheila's book *'This is the Two Week Wait: Real-life experiences of the IVF and assisted fertility treatment two-week wait.* Available as an eBook and paperback here: https://books2read.com/u/3yzdAV

Thank you for reading this book

It means a lot to all of us who have been involved in this book that we are helping and supporting you, and raising awareness outside of the TTC and loss community.

We would all love to help many more people but there are only a handful of us, and loads of you. Would you help spread the word that this book has been published and is a source of support for those on this roller-coaster journey to parenthood? It's very easy and will take but a moment of your time. You can:

- Share the book on your social media accounts
- If you support infertility or loss clients let them know that this book is a great resource
- Leave a review or rating on the site you downloaded or purchased it from
- Leave a review on Goodreads
- Send us your review and we'll share it on social media (anonymously is fine)
- Let influential people in your community know that the book can help their followers
- Tell healthcare professionals who you work with, and/or who support you, that the book is available and can help

their other clients and raise awareness.

If you have any feedback about the book, or would like to share your story/experience in a future edition, please contact Sheila at sheila@mfsbooks.com

We're very passionate about raising awareness of how common infertility and loss is and to encourage people to talk about their journey. We are hopeful that by sharing our stories, there will be no stigma or shame associated with these topics, which means future generations will feel supported and not alone. If you would like to raise awareness, why don't you gift a paperback copy to a family member or friend, especially if you want them to know what you're going through but find it difficult to tell your own story.

If you're a professional working in a fertility clinic or in your own practice and would like to gift the paperback to your clients, please contact Sheila at the above email address for bulk discount information or eBook subscription rates.

If you have a podcast or need guest posts for your website or blog site, Sheila is always happy to share her story so that it may help others. Just drop her an email.

Sheila has written several other books in her *Fertility Books* series; all collections of true-life stories about the emotional realities when the path to parenthood is a challenge, and her standalone book *My Fertility Book, all the fertility and infertility explanations you will ever need, from A to Z* – please see her website www.mfsbooks.com or the next section for more details.

And finally, the eBook is FREE and by purchasing the paperback, a small donation from each sale is made to an appropriate charity that supports ethnic women who are struggling to conceive.

Wishing you all the very best.

Love Sheila & Yemi xxx

Other Fertility Books by Sheila Lamb

Please visit my website www.mfsbooks.com or Instagram @fertilitybooks for more information

FREE eBook: *The Best Fertility Jargon Buster: The most concise A-Z list of fertility abbreviations and acronyms you will ever need*

Are you confused by the infertility abbreviations used on social media sites? It's like a new language you need to learn at a very stressful time, isn't it? This book is your must-have companion - a comprehensive list of over 250 need-to-know medical and non-medical abbreviations and acronyms, to help you as you navigate this roller-coaster journey.

Sign up to download the FREE eBook here and join my newsletter: https://www.mfsbooks.co.uk

This is Trying To Conceive: real-life experiences dealing with infertility

Infertility sucks doesn't it? You shouldn't feel alone whilst on your journey to having a baby. Read heart-breaking and inspirational stories from the fabulous TTC community, who want to support you and let you know that #youarenotalone.

Available in print and as an eBook here: https://books2read. com/u/bPXw27

This is IVF and Other Fertility Treatments: real-life experiences of going through fertility treatment

Are you currently preparing to do an IVF cycle, or are you about to start another round of fertility treatment? Read honest, emotional short stories from infertility warriors - they have your back and are here whenever you need them, day or night. Further support during fertility treatment can be found in my next book *This is the Two Week Wait*.

Available in print and as an eBook here: https://books2read. com/u/31YVp6

This is the Two Week Wait: real-life experiences of the IVF and assisted fertility treatment two-week wait

Are you about to go through the dreaded two-week wait after fertility treatment? Whether this is your first TWW or you've been here before, this wait has to be one of the hardest times on the journey to becoming a parent. Find comfort from the thirty-plus short, true-life stories. Further support during fertility treatment can be found in my previous book *This is IVF and Other Fertility Treatment*.

Available in print and as an eBook here: https://books2read. com/u/3yzdAV

This is Pregnancy and Baby Loss: real-life experiences from the baby loss community

Losing your baby any time during your pregnancy is devastating, I am so very sorry. This book is a collection of short, true-life stories from women and men who have experienced miscarriages, pregnancy and baby loss and stillbirth. They share their emotions at this traumatic time so you don't feel alone.

Available in print and as an eBook here: https://books2read.com/u/bQdAL

This is Pregnancy After Infertility and Loss: Real-life experiences from the finally pregnant community

Are you finally pregnant after losing your baby, or babies? Are you wondering why you aren't feeling unbridled excitement, luxuriating in your own bubble of happiness? Feeling cautiously optimistic one minute and stricken with anxiety the next? Now imagine having your feelings validated by other women who understand, and who are sharing their experiences in this book. They don't want you to be alone during your long awaited pregnancy.

Available in print and as an eBook.

My Fertility Book; All the fertility and infertility explanations you will ever need, from A to Z

Are you stressed navigating the world of conception? Do you feel overwhelmed by the sheer amount of infertility information available online? This comprehensive, jargon-free book explains over 200+ medical and non-medical terms and includes helpful illustrations.

Available in print and as an eBook here: https://books2read.com/u/mqoNd2

Resources

Below are the biographies and contact details for the contributors who wanted to be listed in case you would like to connect with them. If what they have written resonates with you, I'm sure they would love to hear from you, and please tell them you read their story in this book!

Abbe Meryl Feder is an actress, writer, and producer in Los Angeles. She's an Artist in Residence at the Braid Theater in Santa Monica. Her struggle with infertility led to the podcast 'Maculate Conception,' which ultimately led to co-founding 'InCircle Fertility,' a coaching business helping women and couples navigate infertility. She is also a stylist, and is a recurring contributor to the blog *What's Up Moms*. You can find her way too often on Instagram. She grew up on the mean streets of New York's Upper East Side, graduated from the University of Wisconsin and studied at The American Academy of Dramatic Arts in New York. She is an avid mahjong and card player, an escape room enthusiast, and has been called by many friends a true 'balabusta.' She is married to filmmaker Isaac Feder and they are parents to chaotic and loving miracle twins.

If you would like to connect with Abbe:

Instagram @abbefeder

Podcast adbl.co/ivf

Coaching business www.incirclefertility.com

Aisha Balesaria is an infertility, miscarriage, endometriosis and childfree-after-infertility advocate. She is a Coach and founded her business, mindbodyrevival_coach, after stopping her infertility journey and embracing her new path – living childfree. She now works with others at every stage of their infertility journey and empowers them to create their best lives.

If you would like to connect with Aisha:

Instagram @mindbodyrevival_coach

Website www.mindbodyrevivalcoach.com

Anjulie lost her daughter Summer at 19w+5 days and has also experienced two miscarriages. To help her process her losses she blogs – her blogs are raw, relatable and are helping to raise awareness of the taboo subjects of miscarriage and baby loss.

If you would like to connect with Anjulie:

Instagram @anjulies_mumoirs

Blog www.Mumoirs.co.uk

Email anjuliesmumoirs@gmail.com

Asia Cash is a wife, mother, sister, daughter and friend who has a desire to uplift women and spread joy everywhere she goes. Her contagious energy shines bright in any room, and she loves to encourage imperfect people and help them understand that God can use them in any capacity. Asia Cash is an author, podcast host, and the founder and visionary of The Frutiful Place, Inc, which aims to educate and raise awareness about infertility, and be a voice for those suffering in silence. She enjoys reading and spending time with her family in her free time, and she looks forward to impacting lives all over the world.

If you would like to connect with Asia:

Instagram @thefruitfulplace
Website www.thefruitfulplace.com
Email thefruitfulplace@gmail.com

Chi is based in London, UK. She says "I've travelled quite a bit on our journey to try to have a baby, and now understand so much about infertility and how important it has been to advocate for myself on this journey."
If you would like to connect with Chi:
Instagram @makingbabyo__

Crystal-Gayle and Miguel Williams founded 4Damani in October 2018 after experiencing the death of their first child Damani, in the September. After recognising how unmentionable baby loss and grief are in Jamaica, coupled with the lack of support, the cause was established to acknowledge and support grieving parents. The aim of 4Damani is to break the silence and stigma surrounding pregnancy and infant loss in Jamaica by sharing stories so persons know they're not alone. Through their advocacy, in 2019, the Governor General of Jamaica proclaimed October as Pregnancy and Infant Loss Awareness Month in Jamaica, and October 15th as Pregnancy and Infant Loss Remembrance Day.
If you would like to connect with Crystal-Gayle:
Instagram/Twitter/Facebook @4Damani
Website www.4damani.com

Gurinder Mann experienced six miscarriages, and after giving birth to her stillborn daughter Jiya, she traded her corporate career to pursue her true calling as a 'change maker'. She is now a leading baby loss blogger, speaker and life coach. Her mission is to change the narrative around baby loss, particularly in the South Asian community. As a life coach, she helps women who've lost their sense of self to find their true selves and live their best life. Gurinder never gave up hope and her eighth pregnancy resulted in her having her first living daughter, Simran.

If you would like to connect with Gurinder:

Instagram and Facebook @adrugnamedhope

Website www.adrugnamedhope.com

Kajal Pankhania knows that nothing in life can prepare you for the loss of your baby; after all, you never think it's going to happen to you. Kajal says "Having gone through this heart-breaking pain, I understand how lonely it can feel, how it seems as though the dark cloud will never lift, and yet somehow it does. The world keeps on spinning and life sweeps you along until somehow you find yourself starting to live again. The path is thorny, but as you keep walking, the light does begin to touch your life again. Baby loss is a subject that simply isn't spoken about enough, and it's why I started sharing our story, not only to honour my daughter Aurelia, but to break the silence surrounding baby loss and stillbirth. No one ever has to be alone on this journey, and together I truly believe we can make a difference".

If you would like to connect with Kajal:

Instagram @aurelias_wish

Karabo and Jerry Zwane are co-founders of a non-profitable organization called 'Hannah - you are not alone'. 'Hannah' seeks to provide support to those struggling with infertility - to bring awareness about a disease that has left many destitute and stigmatized. The Zwane's struggled to conceive for seven years. They experienced a range of mishaps during their fertility journey, such as an abnormal morphology, four miscarriages, an ectopic pregnancy and two failed attempts of Artificial Insemination. Depression, shame and lose of hope took the best out of them. They are devoted to help couples rise above the shame of infertility.

If you would like to connect with Karabo and Jerry:

Instagram @hannah_youarenotalone

Facebook Hannah - you are not alone

Email Info@hannah.org.za

Website www.Hannah.org.za

Kezia Ashley Okafor, author of *Flipping the Script on Infertility*, is also a fertility mindset coach and infertility counsellor. Kezia supports women struggling with the emotional distress and mental anguish of infertility to find calm and confidence on their journey to motherhood and beyond.

If you would like to connect with Kezia:

Instagram @iamkeziaokafor

Website www.keziaokafor.com

(Dr) Loree Johnson is a Licensed Marriage and Family Therapist (LMFT) and Coach in private practice, with more than twenty-five years of experience as a clinician, educator, and clinical supervisor. Specializing in women's mental health and reproductive health, Dr Loree helps her clients overcome the emotional challenges that come with infertility - including pregnancy loss and emotional trauma. She also helps couples who have become divided by their fertility journey to strengthen their connection. Dr Loree is a clinical fellow of the American

Association for Marriage and Family Therapy and has served on its state and national boards. She is also a member of the American Society for Reproductive Medicine's Mental Health Professionals Group. Dr Loree lives in the Los Angeles area with her husband and toy poodle. In her spare time, she enjoys salsa dancing, traveling, and reading.

If you would like to connect with Dr Loree:

Instagram @drloreejohnson

Manjeet Sahota is mum to two girls and a fitness professional. She says "I have always loved fitness as it helped me recover from PND after my first pregnancy. However, I retrained as a fitness professional after my IVF journey to help other women overcome struggles, depression, mental health issues, and to create a fun, educational, empowering, safe space to not just keep healthy, but meet other women and share knowledge, experiences and journeys. I long to inspire women everywhere to get fit and utilise exercise as their medicine".

If you would like to connect with Manjeet:

Instagram @fitspiration_fitter

Maria Ali is Pakistani born, and raised in Karachi. She's an Art Director, a Makeup Artist, an Endometriosis Survivor and an IVF Warrior. She says "I've done my Bachelors in Fine Arts, specializing in Creative Advertising from American University in Dubai. After working a few years in Advertising, things started feeling monotonous and I wasn't satisfied creatively, which is when I started my journey with makeup and my Instagram blog @mariasinstaglam. After starting my blog, I went on to get my certification as a Makeup Artist and Educator and I haven't looked back since." In August, 2020, she decided to share her story of her own struggles to conceive and how doing IVF affected her physically and mentally, on her Instagram account in the hopes that it could help someone else. She received hundreds of positive comments, many from people who haven't personally experienced infertility or fertility treatments but were grateful to Maria for raising awareness.

If you would like to connect with Maria:

Instagram @mariasinstaglam

Email mariamuzaffarali@gmail.com

Marise Angibeau-Gray is a Full Spectrum and Reproductive Wellness Coach serving New Jersey and parts of New York and Pennsylvania. Marise comes from a career in art and design but felt a calling to birth-work after experiencing three losses at different stages in pregnancy. She was drawn to understanding the beauty of reproduction and its complexities. She says "What I gained through my healing was a passion for understanding fertility, birth, parenthood and the struggle of infertility that so many people experience in silence, while trying to build families. No one should ever feel isolated in their journey. We all need support, kindness, and advocacy".

If you would like to connect with Marise:

Instagram @4memphys and @fertilityforus

Website www.4memphys.com

Monique Farook is a stay-at-home Mom, wife, and podcaster. Before mom-life, Monique worked alongside her husband as a takeout restaurant owner for six years. She resides with her family in the Washington D.C. metro area of the US.

If you would like to connect with Monique:

Instagram @infertilityandmepodcast

Website www.infertilityandmepodcast.com

Podcast 'Infertilityandme' Schedule to be a guest here 60min-pod

Mysurrogatetwins offers surrogacy services in Nigeria, and was founded following her own infertility and loss journey, after her twin daughters, Myra and Myla, were born using a surrogate.

If you would like to connect:

Instagram @mysurrogatetwins

Nadine Gerin and her husband have been struggling with infertility for over five years and have been undertaking fertility treatment since 2017. They have had five transfers with only one resulting in a positive pregnancy test which was ectopic. Nadine has a history of endometriosis and adenomyosis. They are currently on their second round of IVF. She is a qualified career coach and is passionate about raising awareness of chronic illness and infertility through social media.

If you would like to connect with Nadine:

Instagram @nadineendoivf

Noni Martins is the host of Unconventional Fertility, a podcast that seeks to break the silence, shame and stigma around unconventional fertility journeys. Noni and her husband have been trying to conceive for four years, and it was close to the three-year mark that they found that they had male factor infertility and that they would need IVF. As well as sharing her own unconventional fertility story, Noni hosts other Black women with their own stories, and professionals in the fertility sphere with the hope of bringing more visibility to these hidden stories.

If you would like to connect with Noni:

Instagram @unfertility

Blog www.unfertility.com

Podcast 'Unfertility' on Spotify, Apple Podcasts & Google Podcasts

Ola is an infertility advocate living in Nigeria. She is passionate about creating awareness & facilitating conversations about fertility. Her goal is to destigmatize infertility, make people feel less alone and educate the younger generation about their fertility and importance of their sexual health.

If you would like to connect with Ola:

Instagram @thefertilityconversations and @fertilityconversations

Twitter /Club House @FertilityConvos

Seetal Savla and her husband have been trying to conceive for five years after a diminished ovarian reserve diagnosis. Having experienced a devastating miscarriage and four unsuccessful IVF cycles, she got pregnant on their first donor egg IVF cycle, but sadly suffered a traumatic miscarriage at 9 weeks. The couple are currently taking a break from IVF. Since Mother's Day 2019, Seetal has been documenting her ongoing journey on her blog (www.savlafaire.com) and in the media to raise awareness of infertility, destigmatise the subject, particularly among South Asian communities, and support others in similar situations.

If you would like to connect with Seetal:

Instagram @savlafaire

Blog www.savlafaire.com

Shayo O is a trying to conceive woman who uses her medical knowledge to provide much-needed tips and support for women going through infertility, as well as to let women know they don't have to go through this journey alone. She also runs a page on Instagram and Twitter where she discusses infertility related issues.

If you would like to connect with Shayo:

Instagram @naijafertilityhub

Twitter @9jafertilityhub

Email naijafertilityhub@gmail.com

Dr Sierra Bizzell is a secondary infertility survivor, health and fertility coach, master herbalist, birth doula, and lactation educator. She's happily married to Odell Bizzell and they have three children that are home-schooled. A graduate of NC State University, she received a B.A. in Psychology. Furthering her education at Liberty University, she received both an M.A. and EdS and she recently finished a PhD in Christian Leadership. In 2019, she founded 'Faithfully Fertile Foundation' which is an organization that provides education and grants to those who would like to start their families through reproductive assistance and adoption. She is also the author of two books and loves helping people overcome their health and fertility challenges. Sierra wants to inspire others with her story and she aspires to become a midwife who will one day change the way that people see birth, womb health and fertility.

If you would like to connect with Sierra:

Instagram @ultimatefertilityconsultant

TJ Peyten is a Georgia (USA) native with a mission to raise awareness about Male Factor Infertility. TJ's infertility journey started in 2013 when, after five years of marriage, it was discovered that her husband was the factor in their inability to conceive. Frustrated at the lack of support and resources available for those struggling with male infertility, she used her journal as an outlet to deal with the pain. After several years of coping with their infertility through her journal, she finally got the courage to share her story with the world through her book *Semen Secrets: Truths and Confessions of a Wife's Journey Through Male Infertility.* Their journey to parenthood wasn't easy, but in 2019, TJ and her husband were blessed to finally realize their dream of becoming parents to a beautiful baby girl.

If you would like to connect with TJ:

Instagram @tjpeyten and @semensecrets

Email tjpeyten@gmail.com

Website www.semensecrets.com

www.ingramcontent.com/pod-product-compliance
Lightning Source LLC
Chambersburg PA
CBHW062134020426
42335CB00013B/1215